Royal Society of Medicine
International Congress and Symposium Series

Number 6

Diflunisal: New Perspectives in Analgesia

Proceedings of a Symposium held by Merck Sharp and Dohme in Montreal, Canada on 26 August 1978.

Royal Society of Medicine
International Congress and Symposium Series

Number 6

Diflunisal: New Perspectives in Analgesia

Edited by
E. C. HUSKISSON and A. D. S. CALDWELL

1979

Published Jointly by
THE ROYAL SOCIETY OF MEDICINE
1 Wimpole Street, London

ACADEMIC PRESS
London

GRUNE & STRATTON
New York

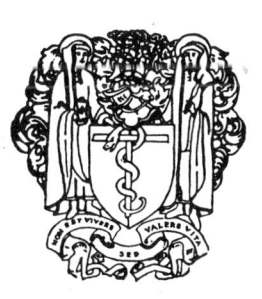

ROYAL SOCIETY OF MEDICINE
1 Wimpole Street, London W1M 8AE

QV 95
D 54
1978

ACADEMIC PRESS INC. (LONDON) LTD.
24/28 Oval Road, London NW1 7DX

United States Edition published and distributed by
GRUNE & STRATTON INC.
111 Fifth Avenue, New York, New York 10013

Copyright © 1979 by

ROYAL SOCIETY OF MEDICINE and
ACADEMIC PRESS INC. (LONDON) LTD.

All rights reserved. No part of this book may be reproduced in any form by photostat, microfilm, or any other means, without written permission from the publishers.

This publication is copyright under the Berne Convention and the International Copyright Convention. All rights reserved. Apart from any fair dealing under the UK Copyright Act 1956, Part 1, Section 7, no part of this publication may be reproduced, stored in a retrieval system or transmitted in any form or by any means without the prior permission of the Honorary Editors, Royal Society of Medicine.

The sponsors of this Symposium are responsible for both the scientific and literary content of this publication. The Royal Society of Medicine has only sought to assure itself of the medical and scientific reputability of the work reported. The views expressed are not necessarily those of the Society. Distribution has been in accordance with the wishes of the sponsors but a copy is available free of charge to any Fellow of the Society.

Library of Congress Catalog Card Number: 79-50308
ISBN (Academic Press): 0-12-792088-9
ISBN (Grune & Stratton): 0-8089-1184-8

Printed in Great Britain by Staples Printers Rochester Limited at The Stanhope Press.

Contributors

A. Andrew
    Clinical Pharmacology Department, Merck Sharp & Dohme Research Laboratories, Merck & Co., Inc., P.O. Box 2000, Rahway, New Jersey 07065, USA

A. Axler
    Department of Orthopaedic Surgery, St. Clarea Hospital, Rotterdam, Netherlands

J. Azanza
    Department of Clinical Pharmacology, University of Navarre Medical School Clinic, Spain

G. Baudinet
    Department of Pharmacology, University of Liege, Liege, Belgium

J. L. Bequiristain
    Orthopaedic Surgery and Traumatology Department, University of Navarre Medical School Clinic, Spain

P. Bernett
    Munich, West Germany

H. L. F. Brom
    Surgical Department, University Hospital, Leiden, Netherlands

J. Christodoulopoulos
    Metaxas Memorial Hospital for Cancer, Piraeus, Greece

V. J. Cirillo
    Clinical Pharmacology Department, Merck Sharp & Dohme Research Laboratories, Merck & Co., Inc., P.O. Box 2000, Rahway, New Jersey 07065, USA

J. Debeyre
    Department of Orthopaedic Surgery, Henri Mondor, Creteil, France

D. Delapierre
    Department of Pharmacology, University of Liege, Liege, Belgium

M. Delgado
    Institut Gustave Roussy, 94800 Villejuif, France

A. Dresse
    Department of Pharmacology, University of Liege, Liege, Belgium

P. Edman
    Department of Pharmacology, Faculty of Pharmacy, University of Uppsala, Biomedical Centre, Box 573, S-751 23, Uppsala, Sweden

A. Eekman
    Department of Pharmacology, Faculty of Pharmacy, University of Uppsala, Biomedical Centre, Box 573, S-751 23, Uppsala, Sweden

D. C. Gengos
    Clinical Pharmacology Department, Merck Sharp & Dohme Research Laboratories, Merck & Co., Inc., P.O. Box 2000, Rahway, New Jersey 07065, USA

Contributors

D. Goutallier — Department of Orthopaedic Surgery, Henri Mondor, Creteil, France

M. Hayat — Institut Gustave Roussy, 94800 Villejuif, France

B. Hazleman — Addenbrookes Hospital, Cambridge, England

W. F. Hoffman — Clinical Pharmacology Department, Merck Sharp & Dohme Research Laboratories, Merck & Co., Inc., P.O. Box 2000, Rahway, New Jersey 07065, USA

G. Holzgartner — Erding, West Germany

J. Honorato — Department of Clinical Pharmacology, University of Navarre Medical School Clinic, Spain

E. Houssianakou — Metaxas Memorial Hospital for Cancer, Piraeus, Greece

E. C. Huskisson — St. Bartholomew's Hospital, London, England

V. Jaegemann — Untere Hauptstrasse, 8050 Freising, West Germany

A. Jaffe — Bournemouth, England

B. Lindstrom — National Board of Health and Welfare, Department of Drugs, Division of Clinical Drug Trials, Box S-751 23, Uppsala, Sweden

R. Marti Masso — Department of Clinical Pharmacology, University of Navarre Medical School Clinic, Spain

L. Paalzow — Department of Pharmacology, Faculty of Pharmacy, University of Uppsala, Biomedical Centre, Box 573, S-751 23, Uppsala, Sweden

S. Peixoto — Gynaecology Clinic of the University of Sao Paulo, Medical School, Sao Paulo, Brazil

J. K. Petersen — Department of Oral Surgery, The Royal Dental College, Aarhus, Denmark

P. Primbs — Munich, West Germany

A. R. Rhymer — Clinical Pharmacology Department, Merck Sharp & Dohme Research Laboratories, Merck & Co., Inc., P.O. Box 2000, Rahway, New Jersey 07065, USA

C. A. Salvatore — Gynaecology Clinic of the University of Sao Paulo, Medical School, Sao Paulo, Brazil

M. B. Santinho — Gynaecology Clinic of the University of Sao Paulo, Medical School, Sao Paulo, Brazil

P. J. De Schepper — Department of Pharmacology, University of Leuven, Leuven, Belgium

S. L. Steelman — Clinical Pharmacology Department, Merck Sharp & Dohme Research Laboratories, Merck & Co., Inc., P.O. Box 2000, Rahway, New Jersey 07065, USA

K. F. Tempero — Clinical Pharmacology Department, Merck Sharp & Dohme Research Laboratories, Merck & Co., Inc., P.O. Box 2000, Rahway, New Jersey 07065, USA

T. B. Tjandramaga — Department of Pharmacology, University of Leuven, Leuven, Belgium

J. R. Valenti — Orthopaedic Surgery and Traumatology Department University of Navarre Medical School Clinic, Spain

V. Ventafridda
  Italy

Acknowledgement

Members of the Merck, Sharp and Dohme Research Laboratories Clinical Research Group made important contributions to the studies presented at this symposium

Piero Angeletti M.D.
  Italy
Francois Bock M.D.
  France
Hans Braun M.D.
  Germany
Al Getson M.S.
  USA
Alec Kahn M.D.
  Holland
Krister Kristiansen Ph.D.
  Sweden
Ronald Kramp M.D., Ph.D.
  Belgium
Rasik Ranchhod M.D.
  Spain
Peter Roylance M.D.
  United Kingdom
Cid Godoy M.D.
  Brazil
Basil Seitanides M.D.
  Greece
Cornelius van Winzum M.D.
  USA

Contents

Diflunisal: chemistry, toxicology, experimental and human pharmacology
K. F. TEMPERO, V. J. CIRILLO and S. L. STEELMAN 1

Pharmacokinetics of oral diflunisal
A. DRESSE, D. DELAPIERRE and G. BAUDINET 21

The activity of diflunisal and dextropropoxiphene on experimental pain in man
L. PAALZOW, P. EDMAN, A. EEKMAN and B. LINDSTROM . . 27

Clinical experience with thermography using diflunisal in the rheumatic diseases
B. HAZLEMAN 39

Clinical reports
(1) **Diflunisal compared with placebo in acute untreated lumbago**
V. JAEGEMANN 45

(2) **Diflunisal versus oxyphenbutazone in the management of pain associated with sprains and strains**
P. BERNETT and P. PRIMBS 51

(3) **Diflunisal compared with acetylsalicylic acid in osteoarthritis**
G. HOLZGARTNER 59

A comparative study of diflunisal and a combination of dextropropoxyphene/paracetamol in sprains and strains
A. JAFFE 65

A comparative clinical trial of diflunisal and glafenine in the control of pain in osteoarthritis
A. AXLER 71

contents

Double blind study of diflunisal compared with aspirin in arthrosis of the hip and/or knees: comparison of analgesia
J. HONORATO, R. MARTI MASSO, J. AZANZA, J. R. VALENTI and
J. L. BEQUIRISTAIN 80

Diflunisal in minor surgery
H. L. F. BROM 92

The analgesic and anti-inflammatory efficacy of diflunisal compared with codeine following removal of impacted third molars
J. K. PETERSEN 97

Analgesic effect of diflunisal in perineorrhaphy
S. PEIXOTO, M. B. SANTINHO and C. A. SALVATORE . . 111

Diflunisal compared with pentazocine in the relief of pain following knee surgery
D. GOUTALLIER and J. DEBEYRE 117

Diflunisal compared with glafenine in pain associated with carcinoma
J. CHRISTODOULOPOULOS and E. HOUSSIANAKOU . . . 125

Diflunisal compared with pentazocine in cancer pain
M. HAYAT and M. DELGADE 131

Diflunisal in the treatment of cancer pain
ITALIAN COMMITTEE FOR THE STUDY AND TREATMENT OF CANCER PAIN 138

Effect of twice daily diflunisal on gastrointestinal blood loss
P. J. De SCHEPPER and T. B. TJANDRAMAGA 141

Diflunisal in general practice
E. C. HUSKISSON 147

Diflunisal: long-term efficacy and safety in geriatric patients
D. C. GENGOS, A. ANDREW, W. F. HOFFMAN and A. R. RHYMER . 151

The current status of diflunisal
E. C. HUSKISSON 163

Diflunisal: Chemistry, Toxicology Experimental and Human Pharmacology

K. F. TEMPERO, V. J. CIRILLO and S. L. STEELMAN

Clinical Pharmacology Department
Merck Sharp & Dohme Research Laboratories
Rahway, New Jersey, USA

Salicylates have been used therapeutically for more than a century, and acetylsalicylic acid (ASA) still serves as the standard against which analgesics and nonsteroidal, anti-inflammatory agents are measured. The short duration of action of ASA, coupled with a high incidence of exasperating side-effects, such as tinnitus, inhibition of platelet aggregation and gastrointestinal intolerance, has stimulated immense research efforts to develop an improved analgesic/anti-inflammatory agent in the salicylate class.

For the past three decades, the Merck Sharp & Dohme Research Laboratories have been leaders in the development of new drugs useful in treating patients with rheumatic and arthritic diseases. Our basic research programmes have resulted in the production of an impressive list of steroidal (cortisone, hydrocortisone, dexamethasone) and nonsteroidal (indomethacin and sulindac) anti-inflammatory drugs. One synthetic research effort had as its purpose the improvement of the therapeutic index of ASA. Diflunisal (Dolobid ®), the nonproprietary name for 2′,4′-difluoro-4-hydroxy-3-biphenylcarboxylic acid (Fig. 1), was selected as a drug candidate from more than

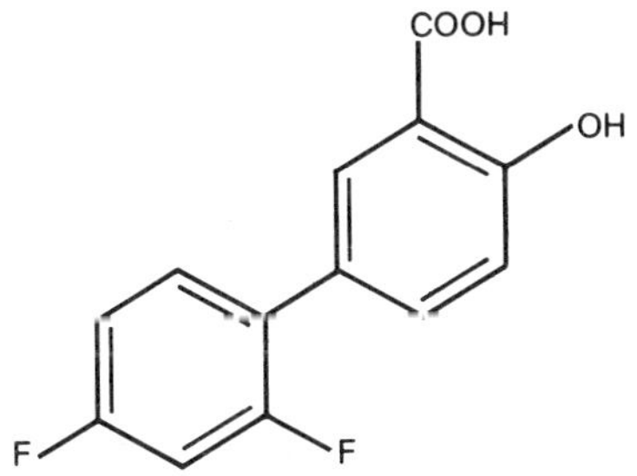

Figure 1. The chemical structure of diflunisal.

500 compounds synthesized for this programme (Hannah *et al.*, 1977).

Both *in vitro* and *in vivo* data indicate that diflunisal is an inhibitor of prostglandin synthesis (Shen *et al.*, 1974; Steelman *et al.*, 1976; Majerus and Stanford, 1977;

Diflunisal: Royal Society of Medicine International Congress and Symposium Series No. 6, published jointly by Academic Press Inc. (London) Ltd., and the Royal Society of Medicine.

Kuehl and Egan, 1978). However, in contrast to ASA and indomethacin, which act only at the cyclo-oxygenase step, diflunisal appears to act at more than one site in the synthetic pathway (Kuehl and Egan, 1978).

Diflunisal has been evaluated in most of the standard pharmacological assays used for the assessment of analgesic, anti-pyretic and anti-inflammatory activity (Stone et al., 1977). The activities of diflunisal relative to ASA have been summarized (Table 1).

Table 1

A summary of the potencies of diflunisal relative to ASA in various pharmacological test systems

Biological Activity	Species	Potency Relative to ASA[a]
Analgesic	Rat	10[b]
	Dog	3[b]
Anti-inflammatory	Rat	8–12[b]
Anti-pyretic	Rat	1·5–3

[a] Assumed potency of 1.
[b] Duration of activity longer than ASA.

In the animal assays employed, diflunisal proved to be appreciably more potent as an analgesic agent (on an mg basis) than ASA. Although the analgesia produced by diflunisal was of the same magnitude as that produced by ASA, diflunisal appeared to have a longer duration of action.

In specific, acute studies to assess the ability of diflunisal to produce gastrointestinal irritation, diflunisal was found to be approximately equipotent to, if not slightly less potent than, ASA. The major multiple dose toxicological studies carried out with diflunisal are summarized in Table 2. No unexpected findings were noted. The

Table 2

A codification of various multiple dose toxicological studies performed in animals with diflunisal

Procedure	Species	Dose (mg/kg/day)	Duration
Subacute toxicity[a]	Dog, rat	12·5–100	14 weeks
Chronic toxicity	Dog	10–40	58 weeks
	Rat	10–40	59 weeks
Carcinogenicity	Mouse	10–40	18 months
	Rat	10–40	24 months
Teratogenicity	Mouse	5–45	During gestation
	Rabbit	5–45	During gestation
Mutagenicity	Mouse	5–45	5 days
Acute toxicity	Mouse, rat		
	Rabbit, dog	>1000	Single dose

[a] Compared with ASA.

toxicological profiles of ASA and diflunisal were very similar, and the various effects seen occurred at comparable doses (on an mg basis). Since diflunisal is more potent than ASA, its therapeutic index is, therefore, more favourable.

Pharmacokinetics and metabolism

Single dose kinetics

In the fasting state, diflunisal (in oral doses ranging from 50–500 mg) was well absorbed with peak plasma levels being reached within 2–3 h (Steelman et al., 1975). The presence of food in the stomach slightly delayed, but did not decrease the extent of absorption of diflunisal (Fig. 2).

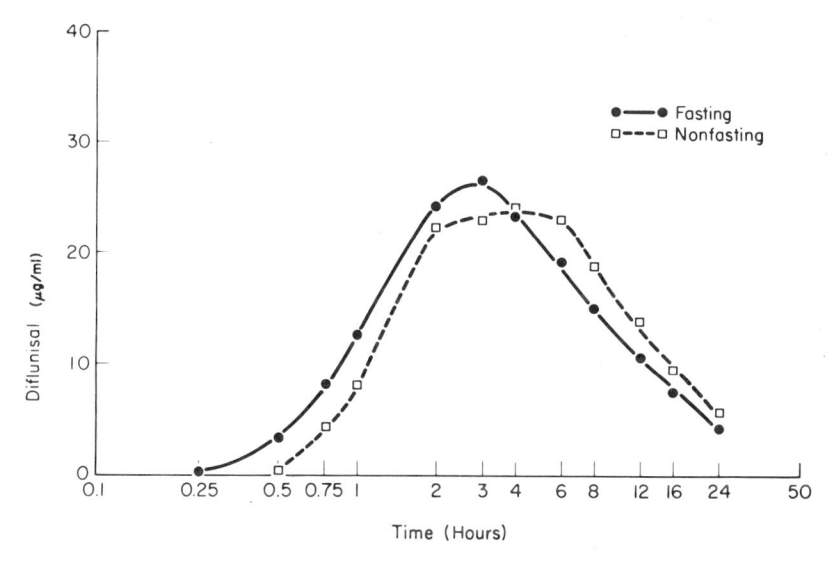

Figure 2. The mean concentrations of diflunisal in plasma obtained from 18 normal male subjects after a single oral dose of diflunisal (250 mg) in fasting and nonfasting states. (From Tempero et al., 1977.)

The initial plasma half-life observed following single oral doses of 125, 250, and 500 mg of diflunisal is dose-dependent, ranging from approximately 7·5 h for the 125 mg dose to 11 h for the 500 mg dose. The terminal slope (determined after plasma drug levels reached approximately 15 μg/ml) indicated a half-life of 7·5–8 h in normal subjects.

In a study employing radiolabelled diflunisal, absorption of the drug from the gastrointestinal tract was virtually complete; approximately 95% of the oral doses were excreted in the urine, with 85–90% appearing as one of two highly soluble glucuronide conjugates. Unlike ASA, diflunisal does not form a glycine conjugate. Diflunisal was not metabolized either by cleavage of the two aromatic rings or by a loss of fluorine atoms (Tocco et al., 1975). About 5% of the dose was recovered in the faeces. Diflunisal has been shown to appear in the bile of rats; however, comparable human data are not available to determine whether the small amount of diflunisal found in the faeces was unabsorbed drug or represented biliary excretion.

Verbeeck et al. (1978) studied the plasma pharmacokinetics of diflunisal in various stages of renal failure, and demonstrated that the plasma half-life of diflunisal increased as the creatinine clearance was reduced. Marked prolongation of the plasma half-life did not occur until renal function was severely compromised (Fig. 3).

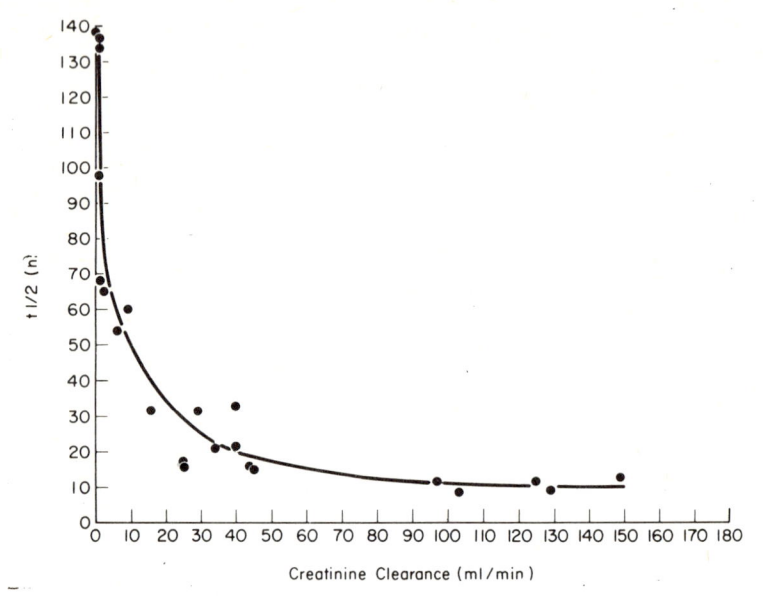

Figu e 3. *The diflunisal plasma half-life (t 1/2), following a single oral 500 mg dose, in five normal subjects and 17 patients with varying degrees of renal impairment. (From Tempero, et al., 1977.)*

Diflunisal is tightly bound to plasma protein (approximately 99%) and haemodialysis is not an efficient means of removal of this drug (Verbeeck et al., 1978). In animals, the rate of excretion of diflunisal can be increased by augmenting the rate of urine flow or by making the urine alkaline (Baer et al., 1978). However, these changes are not of sufficient magnitude to be of any anticipated major clinical significance.

When diflunisal was administered to lactating women, the drug appeared in their milk in concentrations of 2–7% of that simultaneously present in their plasma.

Multiple dose kinetics

The dose-dependent kinetics observed following single doses were confirmed in multiple dose studies in that the time required to reach a steady-state plasma level of diflunisal increased with the dose. A dosage regimen of 125 mg q 12 h produced a plasma steady-state trough level (the trough plasma level is the level immediately prior to the next dose) of 12–13 μg/ml after 3 days. A 250 mg q 12 h dosage regimen required 4–5 days to reach a plasma steady-state trough level of 38–40 μg/ml (Steelman et al., 1975). Data obtained for a 375 mg q 12 h for 4–5 days was consistent with the above in that a steady-state level was not achieved (Fig. 4). Projection of these data indicated that 7–9 days would be required before a plasma steady-state level of 65–75 μg/ml was reached. In a separate study (Dresse, unpublished), the administration of diflunisal (500 mg b.i.d.) to ten subjects produced mean trough levels of approximately 100 μg/ml after 4 days. The steady state-level produced on 500 mg b.i.d. was approximately 110 μg/ml (Fig. 5).

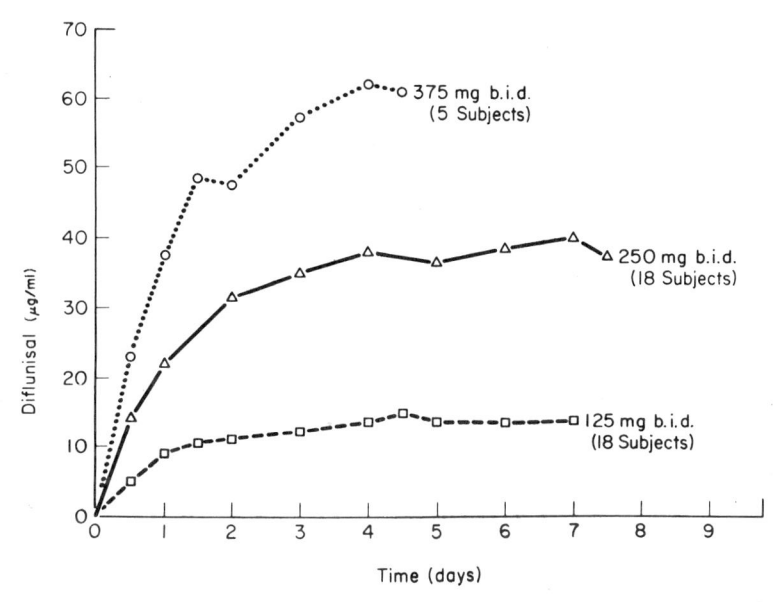

Figure 4. The mean trough concentrations of diflunisal in plasma obtained from normal male subjects on multi-dose regimens of diflunisal. (From Tempero et al., 1977.)

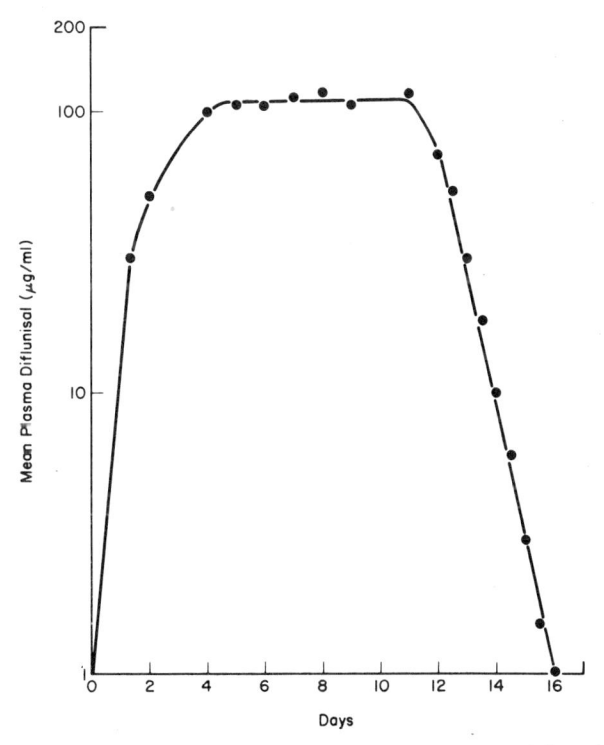

Figure 5. The mean trough concentrations of diflunisal in plasma obtained from 10 normal subjects on diflunisal (500 mg b.i.d.).

The initial plasma half-life for diflunisal following multiple doses of 125 mg, 250 mg, 375 mg, and 500 mg b.i.d. is dose-dependent, ranging from approximately 8 h for the 125 mg b.i.d. dose to 15 h for the 500 mg b.i.d. dose. Consistent with the single-dose data, the terminal phase half-life (determined below approximately 15 µg/ml) was about 7 h.

As measured by trough plasma levels, the administration of diflunisal (250 mg q 12 h) for 21 days did not result in any additional drug accumulation beyond that observed at 5 days.

Pharmacodynamics

General

Various pharmacodynamic characteristics of diflunisal were defined during a series of studies conducted to determine the effect(s) of therapeutic doses of diflunisal on (a) the urinary excretion of a prostaglandin metabolite (7 α-hydroxy-5,11-diketotetranorprostane-1,16-dioic acid), (b) various aspects of uric acid metabolism, (c) platelet function, (d) blood coagulation, and (e) fasting blood glucose.

Urinary prostaglandin excretion

Within 48 h of initiation of a 375 mg q 12 h dosage regimen of diflunisal, the urinary excretion of 7α-hydroxy-5,11-diketotetranorprostane-1,16-dioic acid, the major human urinary metabolite of prostaglandins E_1 and E_2, was decreased by approximately 70% (Steelman et al., 1976). This effect persisted for the 5-day drug treatment period. The magnitude of this decrease was similar to that reported following the administration of either 3g/day of ASA or 200 mg/day of indomethacin (Hamberg, 1972).

Uric acid Excretion

Dosage regimens of either 250 mg or 375 mg diflunisal q 12 h caused an increased renal clearance of uric acid. Serum uric acid levels were significantly decreased by both dosage regimens (Dresse et al., 1978; Tempero et al., 1976). Yu and Gutman (1959) have reported that ASA, at doses of 2 g/day or less, caused uric acid retention while doses of approximately 5 g/day or more exhibited uricosuric activity.

Platelet function

Many nonsteroidal, anti-inflammatory/analgesic agents affect platelet function and blood coagulation, presumably via their inhibitory actions on the enzymes involved in the prostaglandin synthetase system (Hamberg et al., 1974), particularly the formation of thromboxane A_2 (Hamberg et al., 1975). Exposure to ASA impairs the ability of platelets to respond to aggregation stimuli for the life of the platelet, while indomethacin exerts a reversible inhibition of platelet aggregation. The effect of indomethacin disappeared within 12–24 h following termination of indomethacin treatment (Smit-Sibinga et al., 1975). In contrast, diflunisal, in single doses as high as 500 mg and chronic dosage regimens up to and including 500 mg b.i.d., caused no significant alteration in ADP-induced platelet aggregation, platelet disaggregation or prothrombin and bleeding times (Smit-Sibinga et al., 1976; Steelman et al., 1976).

Blood glucose

ASA has been shown to exert a hypoglycaemic effect in both diabetic and nondiabetic individuals (Hecht and Goldner, 1959). Dosage regimens of diflunisal as high as 500 mg b.i.d. did not appear to have any effect on fasting blood glucose levels in normal volunteers or (at 375 mg b.i.d.) in diabetic patients concurrently receiving tolbutamide (McMahon and Ryan, unpublished).

Special Safety Studies

General

The most commonly reported adverse experiences for nonsteroidal, anti-inflammatory/analgesic agents are related to the gastrointestinal tract (Paulus and Whitehouse, 1973). Most agents of this class, when tested at therapeutic doses, have been shown to increase the rate of blood loss via the gastrointestinal tract. Additionally, many patients ingesting high doses of ASA often experience reversible tinnitus (Myers et al., 1965). Such ototoxicity can occur at or below blood levels of drug commonly associated with an optimal therapeutic response.

Gastrointestinal blood loss

Utilizing the standard ^{51}Cr tagged-red-blood-cell technique, a double-blind, crossover study measuring gastrointestinal blood loss was conducted comparing 500 mg/day of diflunisal with an equianalgesic dose of ASA (2·4 g/day).

This dosage regimen of diflunisal did not cause a statistically significant alteration in the rate of gastrointestinal blood loss (Fig. 6), but, the equianalgesic dose of ASA resulted in a significant increase ($P<0·01$) in the rate of blood loss from the second through fifth day of drug therapy. It is of interest to note that during the last 2 days of drug treatment the concomitant ingestion of 120 ml of 40% ethanol during a 1·5 h period enhanced the rate of blood loss observed in the ASA group (De Schepper et al., 1978). These results were subsequently confirmed in a separate study in 12 subjects in which diflunisal (500 mg b.i.d.) was compared to placebo (De Schepper unpublished). Diflunisal did not cause a significant alteration in the rate of gastrointestinal blood loss over a 5-day drug administration period: mean drug-period blood loss for placebo was 1·05 ml/24 h and diflunisal, 0·95 ml/24 h.

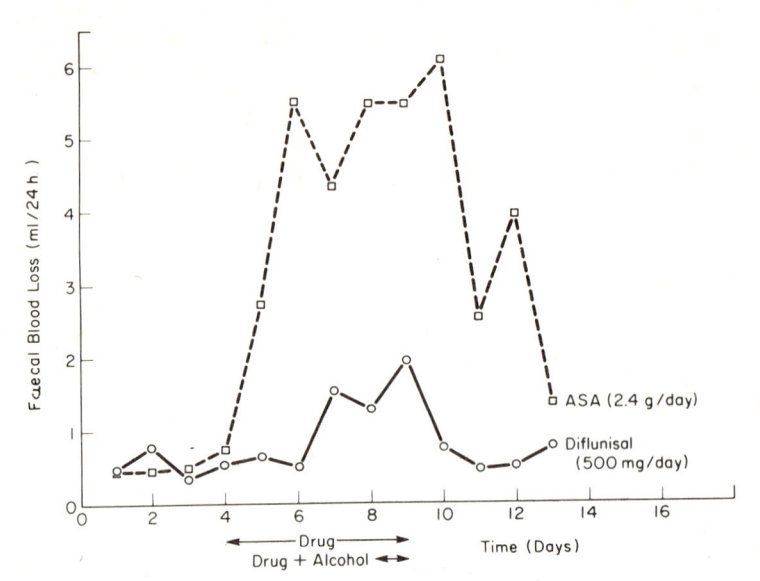

Figure 6. The mean gastrointestinal blood loss experienced by 12 normal male subjects following the administration of equianalgetic doses of ASA and diflunisal. (From Tempero et al., 1977.)

Ototoxicity

A special study of aural function was conducted in which audiometric measurements were made prior to, and 4 days after, the initiation of a 375 mg q 12 h dosage regimen of diflunisal. No complaints of tinnitus were registered, nor were any objective signs of ototoxicity detected (Tempero et al., 1975).

Mild tinnitus was reported by four of 14 subjects who, while on a chronic dosage regimen of diflunisal (250 mg b.i.d.), concomitantly received ASA (600 mg q.i.d.) for 3 days (Perrier, unpublished). The tinnitus was reversible and no objective signs of ototoxicity could be documented by audiometry. None of the 14 subjects experienced tinnitus when diflunisal (250 mg b.i.d.) was given alone or when a dosage regimen of ASA (300 mg q.i.d.) was superimposed on the diflunisal steady-state. No tests were made to determine whether the four subjects experiencing tinnitus while taking both ASA (600 mg q.i.d.) and diflunisal (250 mg b.i.d.) would also have experienced tinnitus on a regimen of ASA (600 mg q.i.d.) alone. Nevertheless, it is to be expected that some individuals taking both drugs concomitantly, at therapeutic dose levels, will experience mild and reversible tinnitus.

Drug Interactions

General

Pharmacological investigations in animals were done to assess the ability of diflunisal to induce hepatic enzymes, and the likelihood of diflunisal interacting with other therapeutic agents.

Studies with male and female albino rats treated for 4 days with diflunisal (10–90 mg/kg/day) indicated that diflunisal was not a strong enzyme inducer. Only the female rats showed a decreased hexobarbital (150 mg/kg) sleeping time. Neither sex showed altered sleeping times when a single dose of diflunisal was given 24 h before hexobarbital was utilized. In contrast, SKF-525A (20 mg/kg), given 60 min before hexobarbital, significantly prolonged the sleeping time for both sexes, and a 1- or 4-day course of phenobarbital (75 mg/kg/day) significantly shortened the sleeping time of both sexes. A single dose of phenobarbital given 60 min before hexobarbital shortened the sleeping time for females but not for males (Tocco et al., 1975).

Drug interaction studies were performed in beagles to determine whether coadministration of diflunisal (in doses up to 10 mg/kg, b.i.d.) would alter the steady-state prothrombin time realised during chronic bishydroxycoumarin therapy or the glucose tolerance curve during chronic tolbutamide administration. Diflunisal did not influence the activity of either drug (Tocco et al., 1975).

In vitro protein-binding studies (MSD, unpublished) using human plasma indicated that diflunisal did not affect the binding of hydrochlorothiazide, warfarin, dicoumarol, digitoxin or indomethacin. However, at maximum therapeutic plasma levels ($\geqslant 100$ μg/ml), diflunisal did displace ASA (11%), and tolbutamide (67%), resulting in higher plasma levels of free drug. None of the above-mentioned drugs interferred with diflunisal binding. Based on plasma binding considerations alone, none of the drugs would be expected to produce a drug interaction in patients on diflunisal therapy. Diflunisal, in contrast, might be expected to produce a drug interaction in patients on ASA or tolbutamide therapy, but, predictions of clinically significant drug interactions based solely on *in vitro* protein-binding data are not always validated. Therefore, studies were done in humans to determine whether diflunisal had clinically meaningful interactions with nonsteroidal, anti-inflammatory/analgesic agents, oral anti-coagulants, thiazide diuretics, and oral anti-diabetic drugs.

Nonsteroidal, anti-inflammatory/analgesic agents

ASA

Diflunisal did not influence the absorption or metabolism of single 600 mg doses of ASA (Schulz and Donath, unpublished). However, data generated by administering ASA (300 mg, single dose and q.i.d.; 600 mg, single dose and q.i.d.) along with diflunisal (250 mg b.i.d.) indicated that only the 600 mg q.i.d. regimen of ASA lowered plasma diflunisal levels during the 3 days in which the drugs were given concomitantly (Ferrier, unpublished). The mean drop in the diflunisal plasma level was approximately 15% and, while statistically significant, is not anticipated to have clinical significance.

Indomethacin

During coadministration of diflunisal (250 mg b.i.d.) and indomethacin (25 mg t.i.d.), an acute increase in plasma concentrations of indomethacin (∼30–35%) was observed (De Schepper, unpublished). Apparently, this rise was due to a decrease in the renal clearance rate of indomethacin. These changes disappeared during a

7-day coadministration period. After one week of coadministration the only significant change from baseline was an increased time to peak plasma level for indomethacin. These interactions are probably not of clinical importance, but this assumption has yet to be verified.

Naproxen

No alterations in naproxen levels in blood and urine were detected when subjects on naproxen (250 mg b.i.d.) also took 250 mg b.i.d. of diflunisal (Dresse, unpublished).

Oral anticoagulants

Acenocoumarol

Three of six individuals stabilized on oral acenocoumarol (range: 1 mg/day to 5 mg/day) experienced decreases in clotting factors II, VII, and X and increases in prothrombin times—all of doubtful clinical significance—after beginning a concomitant regimen of 375 mg b.i.d. of diflunisal (Caruso, unpublished). An acenocoumarol dosage adjustment may be necessary after concomitant therapy with diflunisal has been initiated.

Phenprocoumon

Results from five of seven subjects who received concomitant therapeutic doses of phenprocoumon (range: 0.75 mg/day to 3 mg/day) and diflunisal (375 mg b.i.d.) indicated that there was a statistically significant interaction between these two drugs (Caruso, unpublished; Vermylen, unpublished). The clinical significance, if any, is unknown.

In vitro binding studies (de Schepper, unpublished) with human plasma indicated that therapeutic plasma levels of diflunisal displaced only about 0.1% of protein-bound phenprocoumon. In the same study, therapeutic concentrations of phenylbutazone displaced 10–20 times more phenprocoumon than did the diflunisal.

Warfarin

Pilot information obtained from the study of five patients during concomitant administration of therapeutic doses of warfarin and diflunisal (500 mg b.i.d.) indicated that there was no clinically significant interaction between these two drugs (Breckenridge, unpublished).

Thiazide diuretics (Hydrochlorothiazide)

Concomitant administration of diflunisal (375 mg b.i.d.) and hydrochlorothiazide (50 mg b.i.d.) resulted in a 25–30% increase in the plasma levels of hydrochlorothiazide. This increase was probably secondary to a decrease in the renal excretion of hydrochlorothiazide. Such alteration of plasma hydrochlorothiazide levels is not anticipated to be of any clinical significance, since neither the incidence of side effects nor the therapeutic (diuretic and anti-hypertensive) activity of hydrochlorothiazide increases appreciably when the dosage regimen is raised four-fold (McLeod et al., 1970).

The uricosuric activity of this dosage regimen of diflunisal completely antagonised the uric acid retention seen during hydrochlorothiazide therapy (Tempero et al., 1976).

Oral antidiabetic agents (tolbutamide)

When patients taking tolbutamide (range: 1 g/day to 3 g/day) for control of diabetes mellitus added diflunisal (375 mg b.i.d.) to their daily drug intake, no alterations in blood tolbutamide levels or in fasting glucose levels were detected (McMahon and Ryan, unpublished). It was concluded that no clinically meaningful drug interaction occurred between these drugs at the doses utilized.

Pilot Analgesic Efficacy Trials

In order to determine and correlate the analgesic efficacy and tolerability of various single doses of diflunisal, double-blind clinical trials were run in patients with pain due to episiotomy (Devroey et al., 1977) and orthopedic surgery (Honig et al., 1978). In each study approximately 150 patients who were experiencing moderate to severe pain following the surgical procedure received single doses of 125, 250 or 500 mg of diflunisal, placebo or 600 mg ASA. The degree of pain and pain relief experienced was assessed hourly for 6–8 h following administration of the test drug. The pattern of placebo response indicated that the pain following meniscectomy was more severe than that experienced following episiotomy.

Diflunisal (125 mg and 250 mg) produced significant ($P<0.05$) analgesia according to standard SPID (sum of the pain intensity differences) methodology. However, 500 mg of diflunisal was needed to produce a maximum level of analgesia equal to that produced by 600 mg ASA. The effect of ASA peaked at 3–4 h post-drug administration and then waned. The maximum analgesic activity of diflunisal persisted undiminished throughout the observation period (Figs 7, 8, 9, 10).

These observations, coupled with the long plasma half-life observed during pharmacokinetic studies, led to the evaluation of diflunisal for b.i.d. therapy. To test the adequacy of a b.i.d. regimen, a 2-week, double-blind, placebo-controlled study was performed in 108 patients experiencing pain secondary to osteoarthritis of the hip (Cirillo et al., 1978).

At the end of two weeks, diflunisal (250 mg b.i.d.) proved significantly superior ($P<0.05$) to placebo in all efficacy parameters: weight-bearing pain, night pain, difficulty in a specific functional activity, duration of stiffness, passive motion pain, intermalleolar distance, abduction, overall disease activity, and global assessment of response to drug.

In the patients' opinion 78% of the group taking diflunisal had an excellent or good overall response compared to 46% taking placebo (Table 3). This is a statistically significant difference ($P<0.01$).

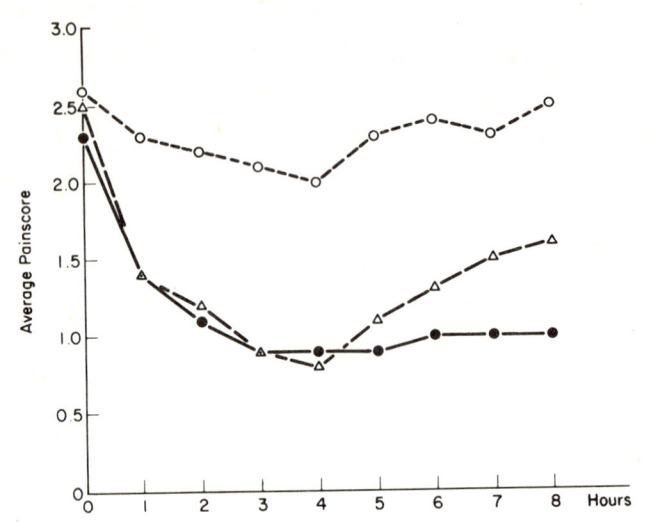

Figure 7. Mean pain scores from patients suffering from post-episiotomy pain. 0 = no pain; 1 = mild pain which is easily tolerated; 2 = moderate pain with continuous awareness of discomfort; 3 = severe pain. ● = Diflunisal, 500 mg single dose (n = 14); △ = ASA, 600 mg single dose (n = 13); ○ = Placebo (n = 15).

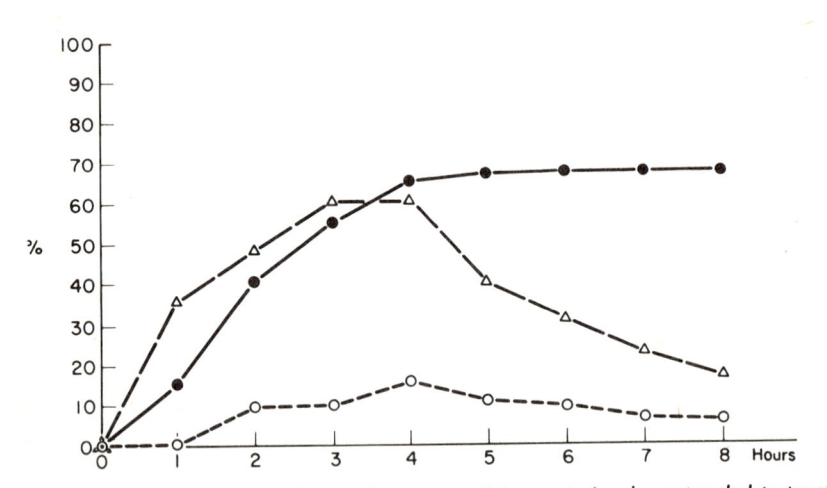

Figure 8. Percentage of patients suffering from post-episiotomy pain who responded to treatment with satisfactory pain relief (decrease in pain score ⩾ 2). ● = Diflunisal, 500 mg single dose; △ = ASA, 600 mg single dose; ○ = Placebo.

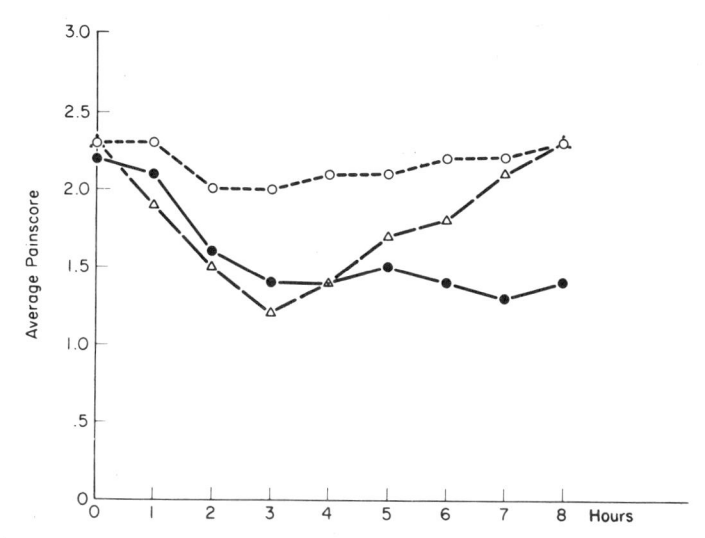

Figure 9. Mean pain scores from patients suffering from post-meniscectomy pain. 0 = no pain; 1 = mild pain which is easily tolerated; 2 = moderate pain with continuous awareness of discomfort; 3 = severe pain. ● = Diflunisal, 500 mg single dose (n = 31); △ = ASA, 600 mg single dose (n = 30); ○ = Placebo (n = 29).

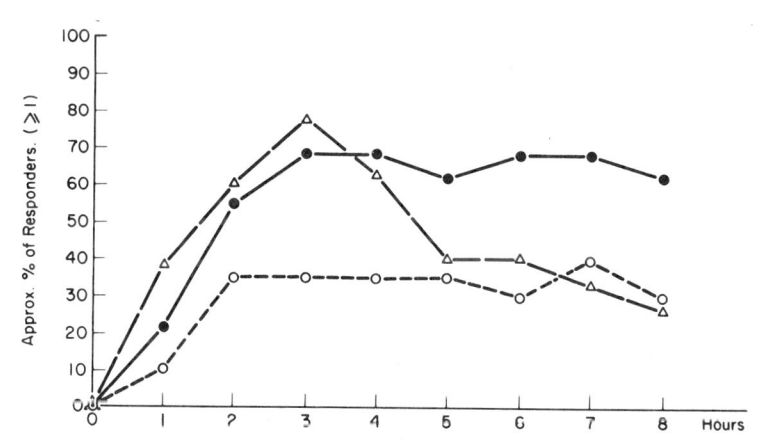

Figure 10. Percentage of patients suffering from post-meniscectomy pain who responded to treatment with satisfactory pain relief. ● = Diflunisal, 500 mg single dose (n = 3); △ = ASA, 600 mg single dose (n = 30); ○ = Placebo (n = 29).

In the investigators' opinion 73% of the patients taking diflunisal had an excellent or good overall response, compared to 40% taking placebo (Table 3). This is also a statistically significant difference ($P<0.01$).

A dose-ranging trial comparing diflunisal (250 mg or 375 mg b.i.d.) with ASA (600 mg or 900 mg q.i.d.) was performed to assess the relative potency of diflunisal when used in a chronic dose regimen (Inberg et al., 1975). The majority of osteoarthritic patients receiving 250 mg diflunisal on a b.i.d. schedule experienced satis-

Table 3

Patient and investigator assessment of overall response to test medication (Week 2) in multi-centre study of patients with pain secondary to osteoarthritis of the hip (from Cirillo et al., 1978.)

Response	Patient Assessment Diflunisal No. Pts.	%	Placebo No. Pts.	%
Excellent	37	72	22	46
Good	3	6	0	0
Fair	7	14	12	25
Poor/None	4	8	14	29
TOTAL	51	100	48	100

Response	Investigator Assessment Diflunisal No. Pts.	%	Placebo No. Pts.	%
Excellent	35	69	19	40
Good	2	4	0	0
Fair	8	15	18	37
Poor/None	6	12	11	23
TOTAL	51	100	48	100

factory pain relief. When the diflunisal dose was raised to 375 mg b.i.d., the percentage of patients experiencing satisfactory pain relief in this small study rose to 100%. Relative potency calculations indicated that, when utilized for chronic therapy, diflunisal appears to be about four times as potent (on a mg basis) as ASA.

Tolerability

During the Phase I and IIa studies reported herein, 398 subjects and patients received single doses of diflunisal ranging from 50–500 mg, and 230 subjects and patients received multiple doses of diflunisal ranging from 125–500 mg b.i.d. for periods up to 21 days. Nine out of the 398 people receiving single doses of diflunisal and 18 of the 230 individuals receiving multiple doses of diflunisal reported mild or moderate adverse experiences which were rated as possibly, probably or definitely drug related. Fourteen of the 27 adverse effects (five out of nine on single doses and nine out of 18 on multiple doses) were gastrointestinal disturbances: nausea, vomiting, epigastric pain, pyrosis and diarrhoea. The low incidence of adverse effects during single dose (2·3%) and multiple dose (7·8%) regimens indicated that diflunisal was well tolerated.

Two subjects developed skin rashes while taking diflunisal (one on 250 mg b.i.d. and one on 375 mg b.i.d.), and their reactions were thought to be drug related (Cirillo et al., 1978; Tempero et al., 1977). Some months later, one of the subjects took an ASA-containing drug and experienced a recurrence of the skin rash. This was interpreted as evidence of cross-sensitivity between diflunisal and ASA (Tempero et al., 1977).

Conclusion

Diflunisal is a novel analgesic agent which is well absorbed following oral administration. It is eliminated, almost completely, via the kidneys as unchanged drug or two soluble glucuronide metabolites. The molecule itself is not metabolized. The drug exhibits dose-related, but predictable, pharmacokinetics. The initial plasma half-life for diflunisal following multiple doses of 125 mg b.i.d. to 500 mg b.i.d. is dose-dependent, ranging from approximately 8 h for the 125 mg b.i.d. dose to 15 h for the 500 mg b.i.d. dose. The terminal plasma half-life is about 7·5 h.

During multiple-dose administration, the time required to achieve steady-state plasma levels varied with the dose. A dosage regimen of 125 mg b.i.d. required 3–4 days, while a regimen of 500 mg b.i.d. required 7–9 days, to approximate a steady-state plasma level.

A dosage regimen of 375 mg diflunisal q 12 h decreased the urinary excretion of the major human prostaglandin E metabolite, 7 α-hydroxy-5,11-diketotetranorprostane-1,16-dioic acid, and all doses anticipated for therapeutic use exhibited significant uricosuric activity. Clinically effective doses did not cause tinnitus, nor significantly alter gastrointestinal blood loss, affect fasting blood glucose, bleeding time, or platelet function.

No clinically important drug interactions with diflunisal have been found to date, although some slight alterations in blood and urine drug levels have been noted. The slight increase in prothrombin time seen when diflunisal and acenocoumarol were coadministered is not considered to be of major clinical importance.

Phase IIa studies, performed in patients experiencing pain secondary to surgical procedures, indicated that a single dose of 500 mg diflunisal produced approximately the same degree of analgesia as 600 mg of ASA. But, the effect of diflunisal lasted much longer than the effect of ASA. Data generated in patients experiencing pain due to osteoarthritis of the hip indicated that the long duration of activity of diflunisal allowed a b.i.d. dosage regimen to be utilized. When used in a chronic regimen, diflunisal appeared to be about four times as potent (on a mg basis) as ASA.

Diflunisal was well tolerated in all the dosage regimens studied.

Acknowledgements

This paper is a review of 37 studies, and many people were involved in the generation of these data. Therefore, we wish to acknowledge the important contributions made by the following individuals:

Dr K. Anderson, Dr G. H. Bessclaar, Dr J. R. Bianchine, Ms A. Buntinx, Dr I. Caruso, Dr R. L. Davis, Mrs F. D. Deluna, Mr R. DeVries, Dr A. Donath, Dr M. Donati, Mr A. E. W. Duncan, Dr F. Ferber, Dr J. Franklin, Mrs V. Gruber, Dr K. C. Kwan, Dr R. Latini, Ms L. Leidy, Dr P. M. Lutterbeck, Dr F. G. McMahon, Dr P. Morselli, Ms B. Reger, Dr J. R. Ryan, Dr J. Vermylen, Mr R. W. Walker, Mr P. E. Wittreich and Dr K. Yeh.

References

Baer, J., Breault, G. and Russo, H. F. (1978). Diflunisal renal clearance in anesthetized dogs: effect of probenecid, urine flow and urine pH. *Arch. Int. Pharmacodyn.* **235**, 204-210.
Breckenridge, A., unpublished observations.
Caruso, I., unpublished observations.

Cirillo, V. J., Bahous, I., Franchimont, P., Baumgartner, H., Van Gemert, J., Lutterbeck, P. M., Hwang, I. and Tempero, K. F. (1978). Diflunisal in the treatment of osteoarthritis of the hip: a double-blind comparison with placebo. *Clin. Trials J.* **15**, 40–48.

De Schepper, P. J., Tjandramaga, T. B., DeRoo, M., Verhaest, L., Daurio, C., Steelman, S. L. and Tempero, K. F. (1978). Gastrointestinal blood loss after diflunisal and after aspirin: effect of ethanol. *Clin. Pharmac. Ther.* **23**, 669–676.

De Schepper, P. J., unpublished observations.

Devroey, P., Steelman, S. L., Caudron, J., Verhaest, L., Besselaar, G. H. and Buntinx, A. (1977). A double-blind, placebo-controlled, single-dose study comparing three dose levels of diflunisal with aspirin and placebo in patients with pain due to episiotomy. *Acta. Ther.* **3**, 205–216.

Dresse, A., Fischer, P., Gerard, M. A., Tempero, K. F., Meisinger, M. A. P., Bolognese, J. A. and Verhaest, L. (1979). Diflunisal: uricosuric properties. *Br. J. Clin. Pharmac.* (in press).

Dresse, A., unpublished observations.

Hamberg, M. (1972). Inhibition of prostaglandin synthesis in man. *Biochem. Biophys. Res. Commun.* **49**, 720–726.

Hamberg, M., Svensson, J., Wakabayashi, T. and Samuelsson, B. (1974). Isolation and structure of two prostaglandin endoperoxides that cause platelet aggregation. *Proc. Natn. Acad. Sci.* **71**, 345–349.

Hamberg, M., Svensson, J. and Samuelsson, B. (1975). Thromboxanes: a new group of biologically active compounds derived from prostaglandin endoperoxides *Proc. Natn. Acad. Sci.* **72**, 2994–2998.

Hannah, J., Ruyle, W. V., Jones, H., Matzuk, A. R., Kelly, K. W., Witzel, B. E., Holtz, W. J., Honser, R. W., Shen, T. Y. and Sarett, L. H. (1977). Discovery of diflunisal. *Br. J. Clin. Pharmac.* **4**, 7S–13S.

Hecht, A. and Goldner, M. G. (1959). Reappraisal of the hypoglycemic action of acetylsalicylate. *Metabolism*, **8**, 418–428.

Honig, W. J., Cremer, C. W. R. J., Manni, J. G., Buntinx, A., Steelman, S. L. and Besselaar, G. H. (1978). A single-dose study comparing the analgesic effects of diflunisal, acetylsalicylic acid, and placebo in pain following meniscectomy. *J. Int. Med. Res.* **6**, 172–179.

Inberg, L., Holopainen, O. and Tempero, K. F. (1975). A double-blind study comparing diflunisal, a novel salicylate, with acetylsalicylic acid (ASA) in the treatment of osteoarthritis of the hip. *Scand. J. Rheumatol.* **4**, Suppl. 8, Abstr. 117.

Kuehl, F. A., Jr and Egan, R. W. (1978). Prostaglandins and related mediators in pain. *In:* "Diflunisal In Clinical Practice" (ed. K. Miehlke), pp. 13–20, Futura Publishing Co., Inc., New York.

Majerus, P. W. and Stanford, N. (1977). Comparative effects of aspirin and diflunisal on prostaglandin synthetase from human platelets and sheep seminal vesicles. *Br. J. Clin. Pharmac.* **4**, 15S–18S.

McLeod, P. J., Ogilvie, R. I. and Ruedy, J. (1970). Effects of large and small doses of hydrochlorothiazide in hypertensive patients. *Clin. Pharmac. Ther.* **11**, 733–739.

McMahon, F. G. and Ryan, J. R., unpublished observations.

Merck, Sharp & Dohme Research Laboratories, *Preclinical Data on Diflunisal*, unpublished.

Myers, E. N., Bernstein, J. M. and Fostiropolous, G. (1965). Salicylate ototoxicity. *New Engl. J. Med.* **273**, 587–590.

Paulus, H. E. and Whitehouse, M. V. (1973). Nonsteroid anti-inflammatory agents. *Ann. Rev. Pharmac.* **13**, 107–125.

Perrier, C. V., unpublished observations.

Schulz, P. and Donath, A., unpublished observations.

Shen, T. Y., Ham, E. A., Cirillo, V. J. and Zanetti, M. (1974). Structure-activity relationship of certain prostaglandin synthetase inhibitors. *In:* "Prostaglandin Synthetase Inhibitors" (eds H. J. Robinson and J. R. Vane), pp. 19–31, Raven Press, New York.

Smit-Sibinga, C. Th., Tempero, K. F. and Breault, G. O. (1975). Effects of indomethacin on platelet function and blood coagulation. *Proc. VIth Int. Congr. Pharmac.*, abstr. no. 616.

Smit Sibinga, C. Th., Tempero, K. F. and Breault, G. O. (1976). Effect of diflunisal, a novel salicylate, on platelet function and blood coagulation. *In:* "Microcirculation" (eds J. Grayson and W. Zingg), Vol. 1, pp. 211–212. New York and London: Plenum Press.

Steelman, S. L., Breault, G. O., Tocco, D., Besselaar, G. H., Tempero, K. F., Lutterbeck, P. M., Perrier, C. V., Gribnau, F. W. and Hinselmann, M. (1975). Pharmacokinetics of MK-647, a novel salicylate. *Clin. Pharmac. Ther.* **17**, 245.

Steelman, S. L., Smit Sibinga, C. Th., Schulz, P., Vandenheuvel, W. J. A. and Tempero, K. F. (1976). The effect of diflunisal on urinary prostaglandin excretion, bleeding time and platelet aggregation in normal human subjects. *Abstr. XIII Int. Congr. Int. Med.*, no. 215.

Stone, C. A., Van Arman, C. G., Lotti, V. J., Minsker, D. H., Risley, E. A., Bagdon, W. J., Bokelman, D. L., Jensen, R. D., Mendlowski, B., Tate, C. L., Peck, H. M., Zwickey, R. E. and McKinney, S. E. (1977). Pharmacology and toxicology of diflunisal. *Br. J. Clin. Pharmac.* **4**, 19S–29S.

Tempero, K. F., Steelman, S. L., Besselaar, G. H., Smit Sibinga, C. Th., De Schepper, P., Tjandramaga, T. B., Dresse, A. and Gribnau, F. W. J. (1975). Special studies on diflunisal, a novel salicylate. *Clin. Res.* **23** (3), 224A.

Tempero, K. F., Franklin, J., Reger, B. and Kappas, A. (1976). The influence of diflunisal, a novel analgesic on serum uric acid and uric acid clearance. *Clin. Res.* **24** (3), 258A.

Tempero, K. F., Cirillo, V. J. and Steelman, S. L. (1977). Diflunisal: A review of pharmacokinetic and pharmacodynamic properties, drug interactions, and special tolerability studies in humans. *Br. J. Clin. Pharmac.* **4**, 31S–36S.

Tocco, D. J., Breault, G. O., Zacchei, A. G., Steelman, S. L. and Perrier, C. V. (1975). Physiological disposition and metabolism of 5-(2',4'-difluorophenyl)salicylic acid, a new salicylate. *Drug Metab. Dispos.* **3**, 453–466.

Verbeeck, R., Tjandramaga, T. B., Mullie, A., Verbesselt, R., Verberckmoes, R. and De Schepper, P. J. (1979). Biotransformation of diflunisal and renal excretion of its glucoronides in renal insufficiency. *Br. J. Clin. Pharmac.* (in press).

Vermylen, J., unpublished observations.

Yu, T. F. and Gutman, A. B. (1959). Study of the paradoxical effects of salicylate in low, intermediate and high dosage on the renal mechanisms for excretion of urate in man. *J. Clin. Invest.* **38**, 1298–1315.

Summary

The novel, long-lasting analgesic diflunisal, (MK-647) 2',4'-difluoro 4 hydroxy-3-biphenylcarboxylic acid, is well absorbed (>95%) after oral administration. Peak plasma levels are realized within 2 h. The highly protein bound (98–99%) molecule is not metabolized and the elimination kinetics are dose related. Initial plasma half-life ranges from about 8 h following a 125 mg dose to about 15–16 h following a 1000 mg dose. The terminal half-life is about 8 h. Diflunisal is 95+% eliminated in the urine (85–90% as highly soluble glucuronide conjugates). Small amounts of diflunisal appear in human milk. Clinical dose regimens of up to 500 mg b.i.d. are uricosuric and cause the urinary excretion of 7 α-hydroxy-5,11-diketotetranorprostane-1,16 dioic acid (prostaglandin E, metabolite) to decrease by about 70%, but are not associated with increased gastrointestinal blood loss or alterations in prothrombin or bleeding times, in platelet function, or blood glucose. Clinically meaningful drug interactions should not be anticipated during concomitant administration with tolbutamide, hydrochlorothiazide, indomethacin, naproxen, acetylsalicylic acid, or warfarin. A mild interaction of undetermined clinical importance may occur during concomitant administration with acenocoumarol.

Zusammenfassung

Das neuartige, langwirkende, analgesische Diflunisal, (MK-647) 2',4'-Difluor-4-Hydroxy-3-Diphensäure, wird nach der oralen Verabreichung gut absorbiert (95%). Spitzenplasmaspiegel werden innerhalb 2 Stunden erreicht. Das hochproteingebundene (98–99%) Molekül wird nicht umgesetzt, und die Ausscheidungskinetik ist dosisbezogen. Die anfängliche Plasma-Halbwertzeit reicht von etwa 8 Stunden nach einer 125-mg-Dosis bis etwa 15–16 Stunden nach einer 1000-mg-Dosis. Die Endhalbwertzeit beträgt etwa 8 Stunden. Diflunisal wird zu 95+% in dem Urin ausgeschieden (85–90% als hochlösliche Glukuronid-Konjugate). Kleine Diflunisalmengen erscheinen in der Frauenmilch. Klinische Dosenverordnungen von bis zu 500 mg zweimal täglich sind urikosurisch und bewirken eine Verminderung der Urinausscheidung von 7 a-Hydroxy-5,11-Diketotetranorprostan-1,16 Dioinsäure (Prostaglandin E, Metabolit) um etwa 60%, sind jedoch nicht mit einem erhöhten gastrointestinalen Blutverlust oder Änderungen in den Prothrombin- oder Blutungszeiten, in der Blutplättchenfunktion oder Blutglukose verbunden. Klinisch bedeutsame Drogenwechselwirkungen während der nebenherlaufenden Verabreichung mit Tolbutamid, Hydrochlorothiazid, Indommethazin, Naproxen, Azetylsalezylsäure, oder Warfarin sollten nicht erwartet werden. Während der nebenherlaufenden Verabreichung mit Acenocoumarol kann eine milde Wechselwirkung von unbestimmter klinischer Bedeutung auftreten.

Resumé

Le diflunisal ou acide 4-hydroxy-2',4'-difluorobiphényle-3-carboxylique (MK-647) est bien absorbé (plus de 95%) après administration par voie orale. La concentration maximale dans le plasma est atteinte en moins de deux heures. La molécule, fortement liée aux protéines (98–99%), n'est pas métabolisée, et la vitesse d'élimination dépend de la dose. La période de demi-valeur initiale dans le plasma va d'environ 8 heures après une dose de 125 mg à environ 15–16 heures après une dose de 100 mg. La période de demi-valeur terminale est d'environ 8 heures. Le diflunisal est éliminé à 95% au moins dans l'urine (85–90% sous forme de combinaisons glucuroniques très solubles). De petites quantités de diflunisal apparaissent dans le lait maternel. Les doses cliniques allant jusqu'à 2×500 mg par jour sont uricosuriques et réduisent d'environ 60% l'excrétion par voie utinaire d'acide 7-α-hydroxy-5, 11-dicocétotétranorprostane-1,16-dioïque (prostaglandine E, métabolite), mais ne sont pas liées à une augmentation des pertes de sang gastro-intestinales, ni à des modifications de la prothrombine ou du temps de saignement, de la fonction des plaquettes, ni du taux de glucose dans le sang. Aucune interaction cliniquement significative n'est à prévoir pendant l'administration simultanée de tolbutamide, d'hydrochlorothiazide, d'indométhacine, de naproxene, d'acide acétylsalicylique, ou de warfarine. Une légère interaction d'importance clinique non déterminée, peut se produire dans l'administration, simultanée d'acénocoumarol.

Sommario

Il diflunisal, il nuovo analgesico di lunga durata, (MK-647) acido 2′,4′-difluoro-4-idrossi-3 bifenilcarbossilico, viene ben assorbito (>95%) dopo somministrazione orale. Si raggiunge il livello di picco nel plasma entro 2 ore. La molecola ad elevato legame proteinico (98–99%) non viene metabolizzata e la cinetica di eliminazione è in relazione alla dose. Il periodo di dimezzamento iniziale della concentrazione nel plasma va da circa 8 ore dopo somministrazione di una dose di 125 mg a circa 15–16 ore con una dose di 1000 mg. Il periodo di dimezzamento finale è di circa 8 ore. Il diflunisal viene eliminato al 95+% con l'urina (85–90% come coniugati di glucoronide altamente solubili). Piccoli quantitativi di diflunisal appaiono pure nel latte umano. Regimi clinici di dosi fino a 500 mg due volte al giorno promuovono l'escrezione di acido urico nell' urina nonchè dell'acido 7 α-idrossi-5,11-dichetotetranorprostano-1,16 dioico (prostaglandina E, metabolite) con diminuzione di circa il 60%, senza però aumento di emorragie gastro-intestinali oppure cambiamenti nel tempo di protrombina e d'emorragia, oppure nella funzione delle piastrine ovvero nel glucosio contenuto nel sangue. Con somministrazione contemporanea di tolbutamide, idroclorotiazide, indometacina, naproxen, acido acetilsalicilico, e warfarin, non si prevedono interazioni di importanza clinica. Con somministrazione contemporanea di acenocoumarol si portà avere una lieve interazione di importanza clinica indeterminata.

Resumen

El nuevo analgésico de acción prolongada, diflunisal, (MK-647) 2′,4′,-difluoro-4-hidroxi/3-bifenil y ácido carboxílico, se absorbe bien en la administración oral. Los níveles plasmáticos máximos se producen en un plazo de dos horas. No se metaboliza la molécula de gran capacidad de combinación proteínica (98 a 99%) y la cinética de eliminación depende de la dosis. La duración media plasmática inicial va desde 8 horas aproximadamente con una dosis de 125 mg hasta alrededor de 15 a 16 horas con una dosis de 1000 mg. La duración media terminal es de unas 8 horas. El diflunisal de elimina en la orina en más de un 95% (85 a 90% como mezclas glucorónidas muy solubles). En la leche humana aparecen pequeñas cantidades de diflunisal. Regímenes de dosificación clínica hasta 500 mg dos veces por día son uricosúricos y hacen que disminuya en un 60% el contenido en la orina de 7 α hidroxi-5,11-dicetotetranorprostano-1,16 y ácido dióico (metabolito de prostaglandina E), pero no van asociados con aumento de pérdida gastrointestinal de sangre o alteraciones en el tiempo de protrombina o de desangre en la función plaquetaria o glucosa sanguínea. No deben preverse reacciones medicamentosas notables en casos clínicos de administración simultánea de tolbutamida, hidroclortiacida, indometacina, naproxen, ácido acetilsalicílico, o warfarin. Puede producirse una reacción leve de importancia clínica indeterminada con la administración simultánea de acenocumarol.

Sumário

O novo analgésico de acção prolongada "diflunisal" (MK-647)—ácido 2′,4′-difloro-4-hidroxi-3-difenilcarboxílico—é bem absorvido (>95%) após administração oral. As concentrações plasmáticas atingem um pico dentro de 2 horas. A molécula, de forte ligação proteínica (98–99%), não é metabolisada, e o comportamento cinético de eliminação está relacionado com a dose. A semi-vida plasmática inicial varia desde cerca de 8 horas após uma dose de 125 mg até cerca de 15–16 horas após uma dose de 1000 mg. A semi-vida terminal é de cerca de 8 horas. O diflunisal é eliminado 95+% na urina (85–90% sob a forma de glucorinetos conjugados solúveis). Pequenas quantidades de diflunisal são detectadas no leite humano. Regimes de dose clínica até 500 mg b.i.d. (duas vezes/dia) são uricossúricos, causando uma diminuição de cerca de 60% da excreção de ácido 7-α-hidroxi-5,11-dicetotetranorprostano-1,16-dióico (prostaglandin E, metabólito), mas não estão associadas com aumento de perdas sanguíneas gastro-intestinais, ou alterações dos tempos de protrombina ou de hemorragia, ou das funções de plaquetas, ou da glucose no sangue. Interacções clìnicamente significativas entre drogas não são de esperar durante a administração concomitante com tolbutamida, hidroclorotiazida, indometacina, naproxeno, ácido acetil-salicílico, ou warfarin. Uma interacção ligeira de indeterminada importância clínica pode ocorrer durante a administração concomitante com acenocoumarol.

Pharmacokinetics of Diflunisal Administered Orally at a Dosage of 500 mg Twice Daily for Ten Days

A. DRESSE, D. DELAPIERRE and G. BAUDINET

Department of Pharmacology, University of Liege, Belgium

Diflunisal (2',4'-difluoro-4-hydroxy-(1,1'-biphenyl)-3-carboxylic acid) is a new analgesic agent structurally related to acetylsalicylic acid (ASA). In animals, it has been shown to be several times more potent than ASA on a weight basis in various anti-inflammatory and analgesic models (Stone et al., 1977). In man, diflunisal is well absorbed from the gastrointestinal tract. At least 80% of a given single dose is excreted within 24 h via the urine (Tocco et al., 1975).

Dosages of 375 mg b.i.d. for up to 6 months and 500 mg b.i.d. during short-term studies have been well tolerated. Previous results suggested that the plasma disappearance rate of diflunisal is not linear for levels greater than 10 μg/ml (Kwan and Yeh, personal communication). Since the dose of diflunisal will probably be ncreased the kinetics of the compound have been studied at a dose of 500 mg b.i.d.

Aim

The objectives of this study were:
(1) to determine the peak plasma level concentration of diflunisal after administration of a single 500 mg oral dose;
(2) to assess the accumulation kinetics after multiple doses (500 mg b.i.d. during 10·5 days);
(3) to follow the plasma and urinary elimination kinetics;
(4) to obtain data on tolerance and safety of diflunisal under these conditions.

Diflunisal: Royal Society of Medicine International Congress and Symposium Series No. 6, published jointly by Academic Press Inc. (London) Ltd., and the Royal Society of Medicine.

Materials and Method

Study design

Ten male volunteers judged to be in good health on the basis of history, physical examination and routine laboratory safety data, entered the study, after giving a written informed consent. The experiment was conducted in accordance with the provisions of the declaration of Helsinki and was divided into three periods.

Day 1. The kinetics of diflunisal, after a single 500 mg dose, were studied. Blood samples were withdrawn at the following times after the first dose: 0 h, 1 h, 1·5 h, 2 h, 2·5 h, 3 h, 4 h, 6 h, 9 h, and 12 h. Urine was collected at the following times: pre-drug sample, 0–2, 2–4, 4–6, 6–9, 9–12 and 12–24 h post-drug.

Day 2 to 10. The steady-state plasma levels were assessed when diflunisal 500 mg had been administered daily at 8 a.m. and 8 p.m. A blood sample was withdrawn daily before the morning dose except on days 3 and 10, and 24-h urine was collected daily. On day 6, multiple blood samples and fractionated urine collections were taken after the morning dose and timed as on day 1.

Day 11 to 16. The elimination kinetics of diflunisal were studied after the final dose had been taken in the morning of day 11. On that day, multiple blood samples and fractionated urine collections were taken as on days 1 and 6. The plasma samples and an aliquot of the daily urine collections were stored at −20°C until the analysis.

Assay

The unconjugated drug was transferred from the acidified plasma to a dichlormethan phase and back-extracted in a pH8 phosphate buffer (0·1 M). The native fluorescence of the substance was measured by means of an Amino–Bowman spectrofluorometer at 318 nm activation and 425 nm emission wavelengths (uncorrected values).

For urine determinations, the assay procedure was identical, except that initially an acid hydrolysis was performed. The fluorescence intensity was proportional to absolute amounts of drug over the range of 0·5 to 50 μg/ml.

Results and Comments

After a single oral dose of 500 mg, the peak plasma level of 87±μg/ml (mean ± standard deviation, N = 10) occurred approximately 2·5 h after drug intake (Fig. 1).

After multiple 500 mg oral doses, 12 hourly, a trend to a steady-state appeared on the fourth day of drug administration with a tendency to a small increase from day 4 to 11. The mean plasma level slightly enhanced from 106 to 123 μg/ml. A statistical analysis of these results confirmed the existence of a slope (F = 16·26). Furthermore, a detailed examination of the individual results clearly shows that a real steady-state is only obtained in four subjects.

The elimination kinetics from day 11 to 16 were not linear for concentrations higher

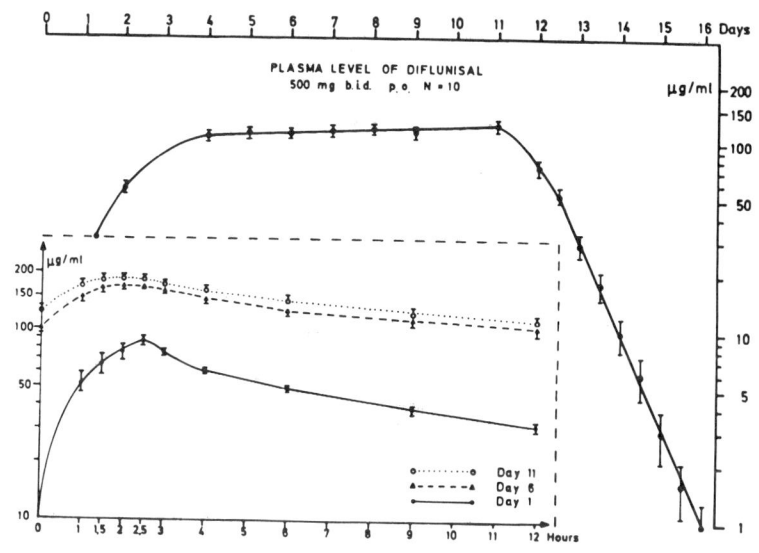

Figure 1. Plasma diflunisal levels following a single oral dose of 500 mg and 500 mg b.i.d. for 11 days.

than 10 µg/ml. At these low concentrations a linear elimination kinetic may be demonstrated with a half-life of 8–10 h. The urinary results confirmed the plasma findings. No adverse clinical symptoms nor abnormal laboratory results occurred under the influence of diflunisal.

The pharmacokinetics of diflunisal, after a multiple oral twice daily 500 mg administration, showed a trend to achieve a steady-state plasma level of approximately 115 µg/ml. The elimination is of the non-linear type for plasma concentrations higher than 10 µg/ml.

References

Steon, C. A., Van Arman, C. G., Lotti, V. J., Minsker, D. H., Risley, E. A., Bagdon, W. J., Bakelman, D. L., Jensen, R. D., Mendlowski, B., Tate, C. L., Peck, H. M., Zwickey, R. E. and McKinney, S. E. (1977). *Brit. J. Clin. Pharmac*, **4**, 195 295

Tocco, D. J., Breault, G. O., Zacchei, A. G., Steelman, S. L. and Perrier, C. V. (1975). *Drug Metabolism and Distribution* **3**, 453–466

Summary

The objectives of the reported study were: 1. to determine the peak plasma level concentration of diflunisal after administration of a single, 500 mg oral dose; 2. to assess the accumulation kinetics after multiple doses (500 mg b.i.d. during 10·5 days), 3. to follow the plasma and urinary elimination after a cessation of administration.

In order to perform these studies, ten healthy male volunteer medical students were selected on the basis of physical examination and routine laboratory evaluation. The protocol of this study is divided into three periods and may be summarized as follows: on day 1, 500 mg of diflunisal was taken by the fasting subjects and ten blood samples were withdrawn at appropriate intervals during the next 12 h. Fractionated urine collections were also retained. That allowed the study of the kinetics for a single administration. Subsequently, 500 mg were administered every 12 h for 10 days. Multiple blood samples were taken on days 6 and 11. A single venous puncture was performed on the other days. An aliquot of the total 24-h urine was also kept. Finally, the blood and urinary concentrations were followed for 5 days after the last administration of the drug. A steady-state plasma level reaching approximately 115 μg/ml was observed from day 5 to day 11. The rate of decline and the other results are discussed in detail.

Zusammenfassung

Die Endziele der Studie waren: 1) die Bestimmung der Spitzen-Plasmaspiegelkonzentration von Diflunisal nach der Verabreichung einer einzigen, oralen 500-mg-Dosis: 2) die Abschätzung der Anhäufungskinetik nach Mehrfachdosen (500 mg zweimal täglich während 10,5 Tagen) und 3) die Verfolgung der Plasma- und Urinausscheidung nach Einstellung der Verabreichung.

Um diese Studien durchzuführen, wurden zehn gesunde, männliche, freiwillige Medizinstudenten auf der Basis einer körperlichen Untersuchung und routinemäßigen Laborauswertung ausgewählt. Das Protokoll dieser Studie ist in drei Zeiträume aufgeteilt und läßt sich wie folgt zusammenfassen: Am Tag Eins wurden 500 mg Diflunisal von den fastenden Versuchspersonen eingenommen, und während der nächsten 12 Stunden wurden in angemessenen Zeitabständen 10 Blutproben entnommen. Fraktionierte Urinsammlungen wurden ebenfalls einbehalten. Damit war es möglich, die Studie der Kinetik für eine einzige Verabreichung vorzunehmen. Anschließend wurden 10 Tage lang alle 12 Stunden 500 mg verabreicht. An den Tagen 6 und 11 wurden Mehrfachblutproben entnommen. An den anderen Tagen wurde eine einzige venöse Punktion durchgeführt. Ein Aliquot des gesamten 24-Stunden-Urins wurde ebenfalls einbehalten. Schließlich wurden die Blut- und Urinkonzentrationen 5 Tage lang nach der letzten Verabreichung der Droge verfolgt. Von Tag 5 bis Tag 11 wurde ein Dauerzustands-Plasmaspiegel beobachtet, der etwa 115 μg/ml erreichte. Die Rückgangsgeschwindigkeit und die anderen Ergebnisse werden eingehend besprochen.

Resumé

Les buts de l'étude décrite étaient: 1°) de déterminer la concentration maximale du diflunisal dans le plasma après administration d'une seule dose de 500 mg par voie orale: 2°) d'établir la cinématique d'accumulation après des doses multiples (500 mg deux fois par jour pendant 10,5 jours); 3°) de suivre l'élimination dans le plasma et l'urine après cessation de l'administration.

Pour mener à bien ces études, on a choisi dix étudiants en médecine volontaires en bonne santé d'après l'examen physique et les essais de laboratoire usuels. Le compte-rendu de cette étude est divisé en trois périodes et peut être résumé comme suit: le premier jour, 500 mg de diflunisal sont absorbés par les sujets à jeun et 10 échantillons de sang sont prélevés à des intervalles appropriés au cours des 12 heures qui suivent. On recueille aussi des échantillons d'urine fractionnés. On peut ainsi étudier la cinématique pour une seule administration. On administre ensuite 500 mg toutes les 12 heures pendant 10 jours. On prélève plusieurs échantillons de sang les 6e et 11e jour. Les autres jours, on fait une seule ponction veineuse. On conserve aussi une partie aliquote de l'urine des 24 heures. Enfin, on suit les concentrations dans le sang et l'urine pendant 5 jours après la dernière administration du médicament. On observe une concentration fixe dans le plasma voisine de 115 μg/ml du 5e au 11e jour. On décrit en détail la vitesse de diminution et les autres résultats.

Sommario

Gli obiettivi dello studio furono: 1) determinare la concentrazione di picco nel plasma del diflunisal dopo somministrazione di una dose orale unica di 500 mg; 2) determinare la cinetica di accumulazione dopo dosi multiple (500 mg due volte al giorno per 10,5 giorni); 3) seguire l'eliminazione dal plasma e urinaria dopo aver terminato la somministrazione.

Per poter effettuare tali studi, in base ad esame fisico e valutazioni da laboratorio, si selezionarono dieci studenti medici, volontari, di sesso maschile, in ottimo stato di salute. Il protocollo del presente studio si suddivide in tre periodi e si può riassumere come segue: al primo giorno, 500 mg di diflunisal vennero somministrati ai soggetti, tenuti a digiuno, a dieci campioni di sangue prelevati ad appropriati intervalli durante le seguenti dodici ore. Si ritennero pure dei campioni di urina frazionata. Ciò consentì lo studio della cinetica con somministrazione di una dose unica. In seguito si somministrarono 500 mg ogni 12 ore per dieci giorni. Ai giorni 6 e 11 si prelevarono dei campioni di sangue multipli. Negli altri giorni si eseguì un'unica puntura venosa. Si ritenne pure una parte dell'urina totale prodotta in 24 ore. Infine si seguì la concentrazione nel sangue e nell'urina per 5 giorni dopo l'ultima somministrazione del medicinale. Dal giorno 5 al giorno 11 una concentrazione nel plasma di stato stazionario di circa 115 μg/ml fu riscontrata. Si discutono dettagliatamente il ritmo di declino e altri risultati.

Resumen

Los objetivos del estudio comentado fueron:
(1) determinar los niveles máximos de concentración plasmática de diflunisal luego de la administración de una dosis oral única de 500 mg;
(2) determinar la cinética de acumulación después de múltiples dosis (500 mg dos veces al día durante 10 días y medio);
(3) observar la eliminación plasmática y urinaria al interrumpir la administración.

Se seleccionaron 10 estudiantes de medicina de sexo masculino y en buen estado de salud como voluntarios sobre la base de un examen físico y exámenes rutinarios de laboratorio. El programa de este estudio se divide en tres periodos y puede resumirse de la manera siguiente: el primer día, los sujetos de experimentación en ayunas tomaron 500 mg de diflunisal y se extrajeron 10 muestras de sangre a intervalos apropiados durante las 12 horas siguientes. También se obtuvieron muestras fraccionadas de orina. Esto permitió estudiar la cinética de una dosis única. A continuación se administraron 500 mg cada 12 horas durante 10 días. El sexto y undécimo días se sacaron múltiples muestras de sangre y los otros días se realizó una sola punción venosa diaria. También se conservó una parte alícuota de toda la orina de 24 horas. Finalmente, se observaron las concentraciones sanguínea y urinaria durante 5 días, luego de la última administración del medicamento. Se observó un nivel plasmático estable que alcanzaba aproximadamente 115 µg/ml desde el quinto al undécimo día. Se analizan detalladamente el índice de eliminación y otros resultados.

Sumário

Os objectivos do estudo relatado eram: 1) determinar o nível de pico no plasma da concentração de diflunisal após administração duma única dose de 500 mg por via ora; 2) avaliar o comportamento cinético de acumulação após doses múltiplas (500 mg duas vezes por dia durante 10,5 dias); 3) examinar o processo de eliminação plasmática e urinária depois de ter cessado a administração.

Para efectuar estes estudos, foram seleccionados dez indivíduos voluntários saudáveis, todos eles estudantes de medicina e do sexo masculino, e tal selecção foi feita à base de exame físico e análises laboratoriais de rotina. O protocolo deste estudo está dividido em três períodos, podendo ser resumido como segue: no primeiro dia, foi administrada uma dose de 500 mg aos pacientes em jejum, e durante as 12 horas seguintes foram extraídas 10 amostras de sangue a intervalos apropriados. Foram retidas também amostras fraccionais de urina. Isto permitiu fazer o estudo do comportamento cinético para uma única administração. Subsequentemente, foram administrados 500 mg de 12 em 12 horas durante 10 dias. No 6° e 11° dias foram colhidas múltiplas amostras de sangue. Nos outros dias foi feita apenas uma única punção venosa. Foi retida também uma parte alíquota da urina total de 24 horas. Finalmente, as concentrações sanguínea e urinária foram seguidas durante 5 dias após a última administração da droga. Um nível regular de concentração plasmática, atingindo aproximadamente 115 µg/ml foi observado desde o 5° até ao 11° dia. A rapidez de declínio progressivo e os outros resultados são discutidos detalhadamente.

The Activity of Diflunisal and Dextropropoxyphene on Experimental Pain in Man: Relationships Between Plasma Levels and Analgesia

L. PAALZOW, P. EDMAN and A. EEKMAN

*Department of Parmacology, Faculty of Pharmacy,
University of Uppsala, Biomedical Centre,
Uppsala, Sweden*

B. LINDSTROM

*National Board of Health and Welfare,
Department of Drugs,
Division of Clinical Drug Trials,
Uppsala, Sweden*

Diflunisal (5-(2,4 difluorophenyl)-salicylic acid is a new derivative of salicylic acid. It has been found to have potential anti-inflammatory and analgesic effects both in animals and humans (Stone *et al.*, 1977). In post-operative pain it has been shown to be effective in 75–85% of patients (Van Winzum and Rodda, 1977). For patients with osteoarthritis, diflusinal was found to be an effective drug and considered to produce less gastrointestinal side-effects than eg. aspirin. In rats, however, aspirin and diflunisal were unable to alter the pain threshold of the vocal response induced by pressure on the normal foot of the animal, although they did so on the inflamed foot (Stone *et al.*, 1977).

Standardized electrical stimulation in animals has been used as a very useful test model for studies of different pain reactions and for the evaluation of the mechanisms of action of analgesic drugs (Paalzow, 1969, 1976, Paalzow and Paalzow 1973, 1974, 1975, 1976), and for studying the relationships between the pharmacokinetics and the pharmacologic activities of several drugs (Paalzow and Paalzow, 1970; Dahlström and Paalzow, 1976, 1978; Dahlström *et al.*, 1978). This experimental animal model has also been found to be useful in humans, and the present study was designed to compare the analgesic activity of diflunisal and one of the more established drugs, dextropropoxyphene. Furthermore, by studying the time course of plasma concentrations of these two drugs it was hoped to establish any possible relationship between plasma concentration and analgesic activity.

Diflunisal: Royal Society of Medicine International Congress and Symposium Series No. 6, published jointly by Academic Press Inc. (London) Ltd., and the Royal Society of Medicine.

Materials and Methods

Three male and three female healthy, non-smoking volunteers (age 22–25 years) gave their written consent to participate in the study. In a double-blind, double-dummy Latin Square study, diflunisal (500 mg), dextropropoxyphene (100 mg) and placebo were given as single oral doses together with 100 ml of water. There was a one-week interval between administrations. The subject took a light standardized breakfast 2 h before the test and blood samples were withdrawn at 0, 0·5, 1·0, 1·5, 2·0, 3·0, 5·0, 8·0 and 24 h after intake. A standardized lunch was given 4 h after drug administration. The plasma samples were stored at −20°C until analysed.

Test for Analgesic Activity

Two electrodes (injection needles diameter 0·90 mm) were applied intracutaneously 10 mm apart in the lateral edge of the volar side of the hand and connected to an electrical stimulator (Grass S88). A single impulse of 1 s duration, consisting of square waves with a frequency of 125/s and a pulse-width of 1·6 m/s was delivered as wanted by the operator. By increasing the voltage in logarithmic steps from 0·5 volt to a maximum of 10 volt the following feelings were registered by the increasing voltage in normal untreated persons (mean threshold ±S.D.):

(1) tickling response (0·86±0·29);
(2) moderate but sharp pain (2·26±1·02);
(3) intensive sharp pain (4·73±2·48).

If the most intensive response required more than 10 volt, the position of the electrodes in the hand was changed to obtain less current intensity for this response. During the pre-tests the subjects learned to recognize the electrically induced pain pattern and the stability and reproducibility of the thresholds are apparent from the section results. The subjects were always unaware of the actual voltage given to them and they only reported to the operator their feeling upon each stimulus when it corresponded to one of the three degrees given above. Following administration of the drugs the three thresholds mentioned above were determined at 0·5, 1·0, 1·5, 2·0, 2·5, 3·0, 3·5, 4·0, 5·0, 6·0 and 8 h. The graded response obtained was expressed for each individual as the percent increase of the thresholds compared to pre-drug threshold.

Analyses of Plasma Levels of the Drugs

Diflunisal

The internal standard (5-(4-fluorophenyl) salicylic acid) was added to the acid plasma samples and extracted with N-heptan according to Tocco et al. (1975). After evaporation under nitrogen the silyl derivative was formed and injected on a Varian 1400 gas-chromatograph with FID. The 6 ft column was packed with 3% XE60 on 80/100 mesh Gas Chrome Q and the injector temperature was 240°, column 190° and detector cell temperature 270°. The gas flows were, nitorgen 30 ml/min, oxygen 250 ml/min and hydrogen 20 ml/min.

Dextropropoxyphene

Dextropropoxyphene was determined by GLC-mas-spectrometric procedure as described by Sullivan et al. (1974), with the exception that d–propoxyphene–2 H_2 (benzyl hydrogens exchanged) was used as internal standard.

Analyses of data

The plasma concentration data were fitted to the biexponential Eq. (1)

$$Cp = A(e^{-K_t} - e^{K-at}) \quad \text{(Eq. 1)}$$

$$A = \frac{FD \cdot Ka}{(Ka-Ke)Vd}$$

with the non-linear least square regression programme NONLIN, run on an IBM 370 computer. Mean values of data points were given the weight of the reciprocal of the coefficient of variation, and individual points, the weight $1/y$. Significance for and between data were obtained by conventional statistical methods such as linear regression, analyses of variance and students t test.

Results

Analgesic activity

Both diflunisal and dextropropoxyphene were able to increase the thresholds for moderate and severe pain after a single oral dose. The most pronounced effects were obtained by using severe pain as an endpoint. The time course of the mean values from five subjects can be seen in Fig. 1. One subject was excluded from the study

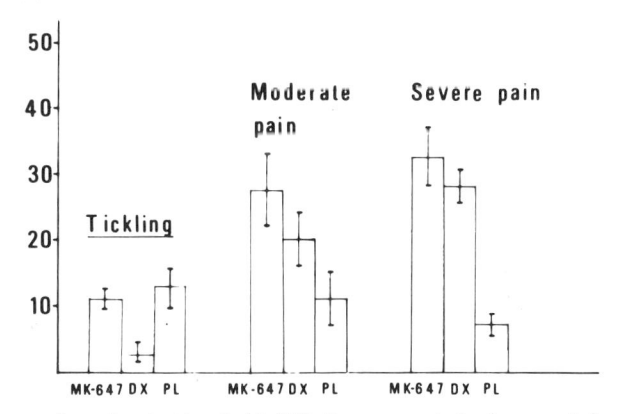

Figure 1. Increase of analgesic threshold (%) for severe pain (mean of five subjects ±S.E. during 5 h). MK–647 = Diflunisal; DX = Dextropropoxyphene; PL = Placebo.

since he missed the placebo. The maximal increase obtained was 52% for diflunisal and 43·5% for dextropropoxyphene. An analyses of variance showed a significant ($P<0.01$) increase of the thresholds for severe pain after dextroproxyphene and diflunisal, compared to placebo, respectively. No significant difference was obtained between the two drugs ($P>0.05$). The mean values of the total effects produced during the 8 h experimental sessions can be seen in Fig. 2. Neither drug altered the

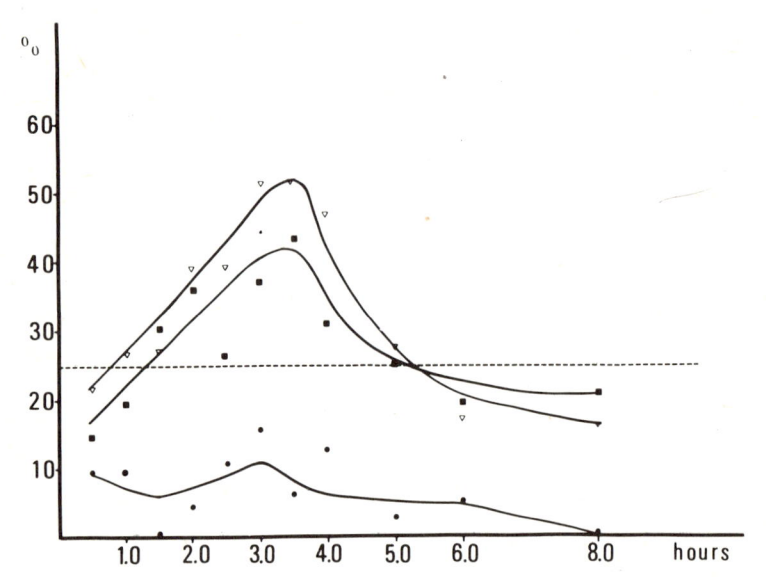

Figure 2. Increase in analgesic threshold for severe pain over an 8 h period (mean of five subjects ± S.E.). ▽ = Diflunisal; ■ = Dextropropoxyphene; ● = Placebo.

threshold for the tickling response and only slightly for moderate pain, but this was significant ($P<0.05$) as compared to placebo only for diflunisal. The thresholds for severe pain were significantly increased after both drugs.

Plasma concentrations profiles

The plasma concentration time course of dextropropoxyphene and diflunisal can be seen in Fig. 3. The data were fitted to the biexponential Eq. (1) and the obtained coefficients and exponents can be seen in Table 1.

The maximum plasma concentration of both drugs was reached at about 3 h after administration. There was no significant difference in the rate of absorption, but diflunisal had a significantly longer half-life of elimination than dextropropoxyphene. However, the limit of sensitivity of the analyses of dextropropoxyphene excluded the possibility of obtaining a slow beta-phase, which has been reported in other studies with a higher dose (Rubin et al., 1973).

There was a significant lag time for diflunisal absorption of about 30 min, while the obtained lag time for dextropropoxyphene was more uncertain again due to the limit of sensitivity of its analyses.

Table 1

Coefficients and exponents (Eq 1) of plasma concentration time course

Drugs	$A \pm SD$	$K_a \pm SD$ h^{-1}	$t_{1/2}K_a \pm SD$ h	$K_e \pm SD$ h^{-1}	$t_{1/2}K_e \pm SD$ h	Lag time $\pm SD$ h	t max h
Dextropropoxyphene	184·6 ± 5·5 ng/ml	0·498 ± 0·055	1·39 ± 0·15	0·282 ± 0·025	2·46 ± 0·22	0·372 ± 0·131	3·0
Range	—	—	0·30–1·94	—	1·92–3·27	0·33–0·96	1·5–4·0
Diflunisal	98·4 ± 23·2 μg/ml	0·641 ± 0·169	1·08 ± 0·28	0·0953 ± 0·0281	7·27 ± 2·14	0·528 ± 0·084	3·0
Range	—	—	0·35–1·82	—	4·53–8·94	0·42–0·76	1·5–5·0

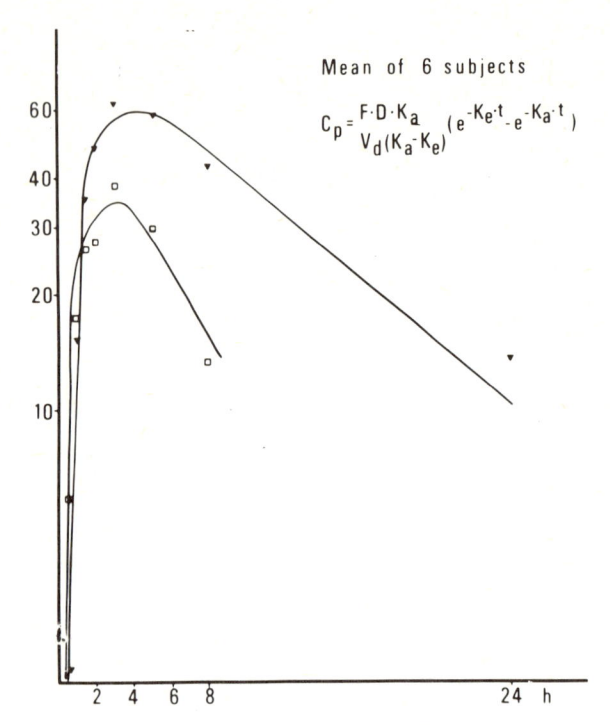

$$C_p = \frac{F \cdot D \cdot K_a}{V_d(K_a - K_e)} (e^{-K_e \cdot t} - e^{-K_a \cdot t})$$

Figure 3. *Plasma concentration time course of diflunisal* ▼ *(μg/ml) and dextropropoxyphene* □ *(ng/ml) (mean of six subjects).*

Relationship between analgesia and plasma levels

The logarithm of the plasma concentrations plotted as a function of the increase of the pain threshold for severe pain at different points of time following the oral administration can be seen in Fig. 4.

The endpoint of effect was considered to be the increase of the thresholds below 25% based upon the experience obtained from animal studies using quantal response (Paalzow, 1969). As can be seen, an acceptable coefficient of correlation was obtained for dextropropoxyphene ($P<0.05$) and diflunisal ($P<0.001$), respectively. The data points are, however, only during the ascending phase of the plasma concentration curves in Fig. 3, since the effects declined quite rapidly below the 25% limit in the post-absorption phase (Fig. 1). Figure 4 suggests that a level of about 20–30 μg/ml dextropropoxyphene is necessary to obtain significant analgesia in this experimental model, while a level of about 40 μg/ml is necessary for diflunisal.

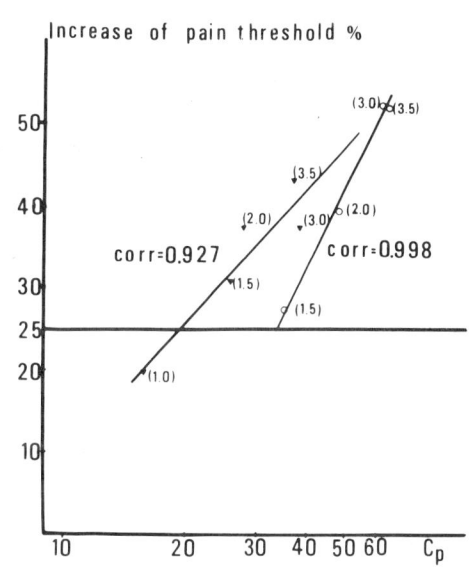

Figure 4. Plasma concentrations (log) as function of increase of pain threshold (%). ▼ Dextropropoxyphene (ng/ml); ○ Diflunisal (μg/ml).

Discussion

The present study has shown that it is possible to demonstrate a significant degree of analgesia to experimental pain after oral administration of a single dose of dextropropoxyphene and diflunisal, respectively. The maximal increase obtained was about 50% compared to the control threshold prior to drug administration. The most pronounced effects were obtained for the severe pain, while no effect was registered against the tickling response. The method of producing experimental pain indicated that it was more easy for the volunteers to recognize the distinction between moderate pain and the severe pain, when they had experienced the latter. Therefore, the different thresholds were always registered by increasing stimulus intensity in logarithmic steps until they had experienced the severe pain. The use of logarithmic increase instead of a fixed numerical step has been discussed earlier (Paalzow, 1969). The ease with which distinct, sharp, severe pain is recognized might explain the more clear effects of the drugs on this threshold.

The plasma concentration-time profiles of the two drugs showed an acceptable relationship between plasma level and analgesia during the ascending phase of plasma concentrations. The duration of analgesia, with a minimum increase of the thresholds of 25%, was about 4 h for the two drugs investigated. The relationships between drug levels and analgesic effects were, however, not possible to evaluate during descending plasma levels, since the effects declined rapidly after 4 h and the reason for this requires further study. Since a single dose of dextropropoxyphene was used it was not possible to evaluate the slow beta-phase of plasma concentrations, which has been found for this drug (Rubin *et al.*, 1973). Such a beta-phase can change the duration of analgesia for this drug and this can be especially evident during repetitive administration (Waife *et al.*, 1975). The correlation obtained between analgesia and plasma levels of the drugs, does not, however, prove that the site of action of dextropropoxyphene and diflunisal is in those tissues which are in instant equilibrium with the plasma. It merely points to the possibility that the rate of absorption is a slower process than the rate of development of the analgesic effects. Another situation will probably be apparent when the two drugs are given by the intravenous route, as has been pointed out for morphine and codeine in animals (Dahlström and Paalzow, 1976; Dahlström et al., 1976; Paalzow and Paalzow, 1970).

The pharmacokinetic profile of diflunisal was similar to earlier reports (Tempero et al., 1977). Since diflunisal is closely related to salicylic acid, which has a dose-dependent pharmacokinetic behaviour, the obtained pharmacokinetic parameters in the present study are probably only valid for the dose used. In other studies of diflunisal the dose-dependent behaviour of diflunisal has been pointed out (Tempero et al., 1977). Repetitive administration of both diflunisal and dextropropoxyphene, respectively, is necessary to evaluate the comparisons of the analgesic efficacy of these two drugs. This is, however, more difficult to perform with the present technique, since it requires that the pre-drug threshold remains stable for a long period of time. The experiment can of course, be performed, but it requires further studies and probably also a larger number of subjects.

References

Dahlström, B. and Paalzow, L. (1976). Pharmacokinetics and analgesia of codeine and its metabolite morphine. *In:* "Opiates and Endogenous Opioid Peptides", pp. 395–398, Elsevier/North Holland, Amsterdam.
Dahlström, B., Paalzow, G. and Paalzow, L. (1975). A pharmacokinetic approach to morphine analgesia and its relation to regional turnover of rat brain catecholamines. *Life Sci.* **17**, 11–16.
Dahlström, B. E., Paalzow, L., Segre, G. and Ågren, A. (1978). Relation between morphine pharmacokinetics and analgesia. *J. Pharm. Biopharm.* **6**, 41–53.
Paalzow, L. (1969). Studies of analgesic and anti-convulsant activity in mice by high frequency electrical stimulation. *Acta Pharm. Suecica* **6**, 227–256.
Paalzow, G. (1976). The potential role of catecholamines in drug induced changes of central pain responses, with special emphasis on morphine effects in the rat. *Acta Univ. Upsal.* **9**, 1–45.
Paalzow, L. and Paalzow, G. (1970). Blood and brain concentration of morphine and its relation to the analgesic activity in mice. *Acta Pharm. Suecica*, **8**, 329–336.
Paalzow, G. and Paalzow, L. (1973). The effects of caffeine and theophylline on nociceptive stimulation in the rat. *Acta Pharm. Toxicol.* **32**, 22–32.
Paalzow, G. and Paalzow, L. (1974). Theophylline increased sensitivity to nociceptive stimulation and regional turnover of rat brain 5-HT, noradrenaline and dopamine. *Acta Pharm. Toxicol.* **34**, 157–173.
Paalzow, G. and Paalzow, L. (1975). Morphine induced inhibition of different pain responses in relation to the regional turnover of rat brain noradrenaline and dopamine. *Psychopharmacologia (Berl.)* **45**, 9.
Paalzow, G. and Paalzow, L. (1976). Clonidine antinociceptive activity: Effects of drugs influencing central monoaminergic and cholinergic mechanisms in the rat. *Naunyn-Schmiedebergs Arch. Pharmacol.* **292**, 119–126.
Rubin, A., Rodda, B. E., Warrick, P., Gruber Jr., C. M. and Ridolfo, A. S. (1973). Interactions of aspirin with non-steroidal antiinflammatory drugs in man. *Arth. Rheum.* **16/5**, 635–645.
Stone, C. A., Van Arman, C. G., Lotti, V. J., Minsker, D. H., Risley, A., Bagdon, W. J., Bokelman, D. L., Jensen, R. D., Mendlowski, B., Tate, C. L., Peck, H. M., Zwickey, R. E. and McKinney, S. E., (1977). Pharmacology and toxicology of Diflunisal. *Br. J. Clin. Pharmac.* **4**, 195–295.

Sullivan, H. R., Emmerson, J. L., Marshall, F. J., Wood, P. G. and McMahon, R. E. (1974). *Drug Metabol. Disp.* **2**, 526.
Tempero, K. F., Civillo, V. J. and Steelman, S. L. (1977). Diflunisal: A review of pharmacokinetic and pharmacodynamic properties, drug interactions, and special tolerability studies in humans. *Brit. J. Clin. Pharmac.* **4**, 315–365.
Tocco, D. J., Breault, G. O., Zacchei, A. G., Steelman, S. L. and Perrier, C. V. (1975). Physiological disposition and metabolism of 5-(2′,4′-difluorophenyl) salicylic acid. A new salicylate. *Drug metab. disposit.* **3**, 453–466.
Van Winzum, C. and Rodda, B. (1977). Diflunisal: Efficacy in postoperative pain. *Brit. J. Clin. Pharmac.* **4**, 395–435.
Waife, S. O., Gruber Jr., C. M., Rodda, B. E. and Nash, J. F. (1975). Problems and solutions to single-dose testing of analgesics: Comparison of propoxyphene, codeine and fenoprefen. *Int. J. Clin. Pharmac.* **12**, 301–304.

Summary

Six healthy volunteers were subjected to electrical stimulation for 1·0 s at voltages ranging from 0·5 to 10·0 via intracutaneous needle electrodes. The threshold for three grades of pain was evaluated before and after 500 mg diflunisal or 100 mg dextropropoxyphene napsylate given as single oral doses in a double-blind crossover manner.

Diflunisal and dextropropoxyphene were both able to increase the thresholds for moderate and severe pain. The most pronounced effects were obtained against the latter pain with a maximum increase of the threshold of 52% and 43·5%, respectively. Both drugs increased the threshold for severe pain significantly compared to placebo ($P<0.01$), but no significant difference was found between the two drugs. No effect was seen on the threshold for the tickling response.

The absorption half-life was 1.08 ± 0.28 h and 1.39 ± 0.15 h for diflunisal and dextropropoxyphene, respectively. Maximal concentration in plasma was obtained 3 h following administration of both drugs. The half-life of diflunisal was 7.27 ± 2.14 h and 2.46 ± 0.22 h for dextropropoxyphene.

A linear relationship was obtained between the logarithm of plasma concentrations of both drugs and the effects on the threshold for severe pain. The data indicated that a minimum plasma level of 20–30 ng/ml dextropropoxyphene is necessary for analgesia and about 40 μg/ml for diflunisal.

Zusammenfassung

Sechs gesunde Freiwillige wurden 1,0 Sekunde bei Spannungen von 0,5 bis 10,0 über intrakutane Nadelelektroden einer elektrischen Stimulation ausgesetzt. Die Grenze für drei Schmerzstufen wurde vor und nach der Verabreichung von 500 mg Diflunisal oder 100 mg Dextropropoxyphennapsylat in Form einer einzigen oralen Dosis nach einer "double-blind crossover"—Methode (= wahllose Methode).

Diflunisal und Dextropropoxyphen waren beide in der Lage, die Grenzen für mäßigen und starken Schmerz zu erhöhen. Die deutlichsten Wirkungen wurden gegen den letztgenannten Schmerz mit einer maximalen Erhöhung der Schmerzgrenze von 52% bzw. 43,5% erzielt. Beide Drogen erhöhten die Grenze für starken Schmerz im Vergleich mit Placebo ($P<0,01$) beträchtlich, jedoch wurde zwischen den beiden Drogen kein bedeutsamer Unterschied festgestellt. Es wurde keine Einwirkung auf die Schwelle für die Kitzelreizbeantwortung verzeichnet.

Die Absorptions-Halbwertzeit betrug $1,08 \pm 0,28$ Std. und $1,39 \pm 0,15$ Std. für Diflunisal bzw. Dextropropoxyphen. Die maximale Konzentration im Plasma wurde

3 Stunden nach der Verabreichung beider Drogen verzeichnet. Die Halbwertzeit von Diflunisal betrug 7,27±2,14 Std. und 2,46±0,22 Std. für Dextropropoxyphen.

Ein lineares Verhältnis wurde zwischen dem Logarithmus von Plasmakonzentrationen beider Drogen und den Auswirkungen auf die Grenze für starken Schmerz verzeichnet. Die Daten wiesen aus, daß ein Mindestplasmaspiegel von 20–30 ng/ml Dextropropoxyphen für Analgesie und etwa 40 µg/ml für Diflunisal erforderlich ist.

Resumé

Six volontaires en bonne santé sont soumis pendant 1,0 s à une stimulation électrique sous 0,5 à 10,0 V au moyen d'aiguilles intracutanées comme électrodes. Le seuil pour trois niveaux de douleur est mesuré avant et après administration de 500 mg de diflunisal ou de 100 mg de napsylate de dextropropoxyphène en une suele dose orale, par essai à double anonymat croisé.

Le diflunisal et le dextropropoxyphène peuvent tous deux élever le seuil de douleur modérée et de douleur aiguë. On obtient les effets les plus marqués contre la douleur aiguë avec des élévations maximales du seuil de 52% et 43,5% respectivement. Les deux médicaments élèvent significativement le seuil de douleur aiguë par comparaison avec un placebo (P<0,01), mais on ne constate aucune différence significative entre les deux médicaments. Aucun effet n'a été observé sur le seuil de réaction au chatouillement.

La période de demi-valeur d'absorption est de 1,08±0,28 h pour le diflunisal, 1,39±0,15 h pour le dextropropoxyphène. La concentration maximale dans le plasma a été obtenue trois heures après l'administration pour les deux médicaments. La période de demi-valeur était de 7,27±2,14 h pour le diflunisal, 2,46±0,22 h pour le dextropropoxyphène.

On obtient une relation linéaire entre le logarithme de la concentration de chaque médicament dans le plasma et l'effet sur le seuil de douleur aiguë. Les résultats montrent qu'une concentration minimale de 20–30 µg/ml de dextropropoxyphène et d'environ 40 µg/ml de diflunisal dans le plasma est nécessaire à l'analgésie.

Sommario

Si sottoposero sei volontari in buono stato di salute a stimoli elettrici di 1,0 s a tensioni da 0,5 a 10,0, tramite elettrodi ad ago intracutanei. Si determinò la soglia per tre gradi di dolore prima e dopo la somministrazione "double-blind" con scambio di una dose orale unica di 500 mg di diflunisal oppure di 100 mg di destropropossifene napsilato.

Sia il diflunisal che il destropropossifene furono in grado di aumentare la soglia di dolori medi ed intensi. Gli effetti più marcati si ottennero con dolori intensi, con un aumento massimo della soglia di rispettivamente 52% e 43,5%. Entrambi i medicamenti aumentano la soglia di dolori forti notevolmente a confronto del placebo (sostanza innocua di controllo) (P<0,01), però non si riscontrò alcuna differenza significativa tra i due farmaci. Non si constatò alcun effetto sulla soglia di "solletico".

Il periodo di demezzamento nell'assorbimento fu di 1,08±0,28 ore e 1,39±0,15 ore rispettivamente per il diflunisal e il destropropossifene. Per entrambi i medicamenti, la concentrazione massima nel plasma si ottenne 3 ore dopo la somministrazione.

Il periodo di dimezzamento del diflunisal fu di 7,27±2,14 ore mentre quello del destropropossifene di 2,46±0,22 ore.

Si ottenne un rapporto lineare tra il logaritmo della concentrazione nel plasma dei due farmaci e l'effetto sulla soglia di dolore intenso. I dati indicano che per l'analgesia è necessaria una concentrazione minima nel plasma di 20–30 µg/ml per il destropropossifene e di circa 40 µg/ml per il diflunisal.

Resumen

Se expuso a 6 voluntarios en buena salud a estimulación elétrica durante un segundo, con voltajes que iban de 0,5 a 10,0, por medio de electrodos intracutáneos de aguja. Se evaluó el umbral para tres grados de dolor antes y después de la administración de 500 mg de diflunisal o 100 mg de napsilato de dextropropoxifeno en dosis oral única de manera cruzada a doble ciego.

Tanto el diflunisal como el dextropropoxifeno aumentaron los umbrales de dolor moderado e intenso. Los efectos más pronunciados se obtuvieron en casos de dolor intenso, con un aumento máximo del umbral del 52% y 43,5%, respectivamente. Ambos medicamentos aumentaron bastante el umbral de dolor intenso con respecto al placebo (P<0,01), pero no se observó apenas diferencia entre los dos medicamentos. Tampoco se observó ningún efecto en cuanto al umbral de reacción a las cosquillas.

La duración media de absorción fue de 1,08±0,28 horas y 1,39±0,15 horas para el diflunisal y el dextropropoxifeno, respectivamente. La máxima concentración plasmática se obtuvo a las 3 horas de la administración de ambos medicamentos. La duración media del diflunisal fue de 7,27±2,14 horas y de 2,46±0,22 horas para el dextropropoxifeno.

Se obtuvo una relación lineal entre el logaritmo de las concentraciones plasmáticas de ambos medicamentos y los efectos sobre el umbral de dolor intenso. Los datos indicaron que se necesita un nivel plasmático mínimo de 20 a 30 ng/ml de dextropropoxifeno para analgesia y alrededor de 40 µg/ml de diflunisal.

Sumário

Seis indivíduos voluntários saudáveis foram submetidos a estímulo eléctrico durante 1,0 s, a voltagens desde 0,5 até 10,0, através de agulhas-eléctrodos inseridas subcutâneamente. O limiar de sensibilidade foi avaliado, para três graus de dor, antes e depois da administração de 500 mg de diflunisal ou 100 mg de napsilato de dextropropoxifeno, sob a forma duma única dose oral e segundo um sistema intercruzado duplamente às cegas.

Verificou-se que tanto o diflunisal como o dextropropoxifeno fizeram aumentar os limiares de sensibilidade a dor moderada e severa. Os efeitos mais pronunciados foram obtidos contra dor severa, com uma subida máxima do limiar de 52% e 43,5% respectivamente. Ambas as drogas aumentaram o limiar contra dor severa significativamente em comparação com um placebo ($P<0,01$), mas não se observou qualquer diferença significativa entre as duas drogas. Não se observou qualquer efeito sobre o limiar da sensação de "formigueiro".

A semi-vida de absorção foi de 1,08±0,28 h e 1,39±0,15 h respectivamente para o diflunisal e o dextropropoxifeno. A concentração máxima no plasma foi obtida 3 horas após administração de ambas as drogas. A semi-vida de acção foi de 7,27±2,14 h para o diflunisal e 2,46±0,22 h para o dextropropoxifeno.

Foi obtida uma correlação linear entre o logaritmo das concentrações plasmáticas (de ambas as drogas) e os efeitos sobre o limiar contra dor severa. Os resultados indicam que para produzir analgesia é necessária uma concentração plasmática mínima de 20–30 μg/ml de dextropropoxifeno e cerca de 40 μg/ml de diflunisal.

Clinical Experience with Thermography using Diflunisal in the Rheumatic Diseases

B. HAZLEMAN

Addenbrookes Hospital, Cambridge, England

Assessment of disease activity is one of the major problems in the rheumatic diseases, and this is particularly true of non-articular rheumatism. A number of indices are available, but most of those in use are subjective, and there is a great need for an objective index of assessment.

Thermography

Modern scanning apparatus can produce a multiple isotherm scan in less than a second, which is conventionally displayed on an oscilloscope screen. The success of any thermographic investigation depends on intelligent interpretation of the thermogram in terms of heat-flow patterns to the skin surface. The integrity of the blood supply to the skin, and the thermal properties and metabolism of tissue, are the principal factors which determine the surface temperature characteristics. The more removed the skin effect becomes from the pathological process, the more difficult becomes interpretation of the thermographic data. However, once the surface temperature variations have led to recognition of a lesion, its site, size and shape can be assessed, and progression or response to treatment can be monitored.

Thermography can be used as a quantitative measure if rigid control of techniques and of environmental conditions are achieved. Factors which must be controlled include the state of the patient, who should not have had recent physiotherapy or strenuous exercise and must remain in a temperature controlled room for a period of at least 15 min before thermography is performed; the time of day must be constant to avoid the intrinsic diurnal variation, and the position of the patient must be standardized for each area.

Diflunisal (Dolobid) has been assessed in the treatment of patients with acute back strain, ankylosing spondylitis, the painful stiff shoulder and in osteoarthrosis. Thermography has been used as one of the methods of assessment.

Acute Back Pain

The efficacy and safety of diflunisal has been compared with placebo in pain associated with acute lumbago. Patients were only included in the study if they had an acute onset of signs and symptoms of less than one week's duration. All patients had a considerable degree of functional disability but no abnormal neurological signs. Physiotherapy was not instituted during the study period which was a double-blind, completely randomized design; the dosage of diflunisal being 500 mg b.i.d. The duration of treatment was 7 days.

This study is still in progress but preliminary results show that eight of the nine patients treated with diflunisal considered that there had been a marked improvement in their symptoms. One patient complained of nausea and discontinued treatment.

Whereas patients with acute back pain often show an asymmetrical paravertebral area of increased heat, the pattern is quite different from the focal area of increased heat seen in lumbar disc disease. Return of the thermogram to a symmetrical pattern coincides with clinical improvement and this was seen with treatment on diflunisal. However, at present it is not known to what extent abnormal patterns can be expected in a normal population or to what degree thermal asymmetry correlates with disease activity.

Ankylosing Spondylitis

The encouraging improvement seen in patients with acute back pain has led to a pilot study of patients with ankylosing spondylitis. Five patients with active ankylosing spondylitis were entered into the study. All were male and were receiving treatment with phenylbutazone, naproxen or indomethacin. Therapy was discontinued for 48 h prior to thermography—all patients had an exacerbation of their symptoms and one recommenced drug therapy. Diflunisal was given at a dose of 500 mg b.i.d. for 14 days and thermography was repeated. All patients reported satisfactory control of their symptoms on diflunisal, and considered the drug more effective (three patients) or as effective (two patients) as their previous therapy. All showed a fall in temperature on the drug, which was most marked over the thoracic vertebrae (Plates 1a and 1b).

"Osteoarthrosis"

Recent evidence has suggested that an inflammatory process is involved in the degenerative joint disease commonly labelled osteoarthrosis. Thermography on patients with osteoarthrosis of the knee has demonstrated that joint temperatures were significantly higher than in normal controls but significantly lower than in a random group of rheumatoid patients. The swollen joints were hotter than the equivalent non-swollen joints. Treatment with diflunisal resulted in a fall in joint temperature and provided a satisfactory control of joint. Symptoms in five patients treated with diflunisal (Plates 2a and 2b).

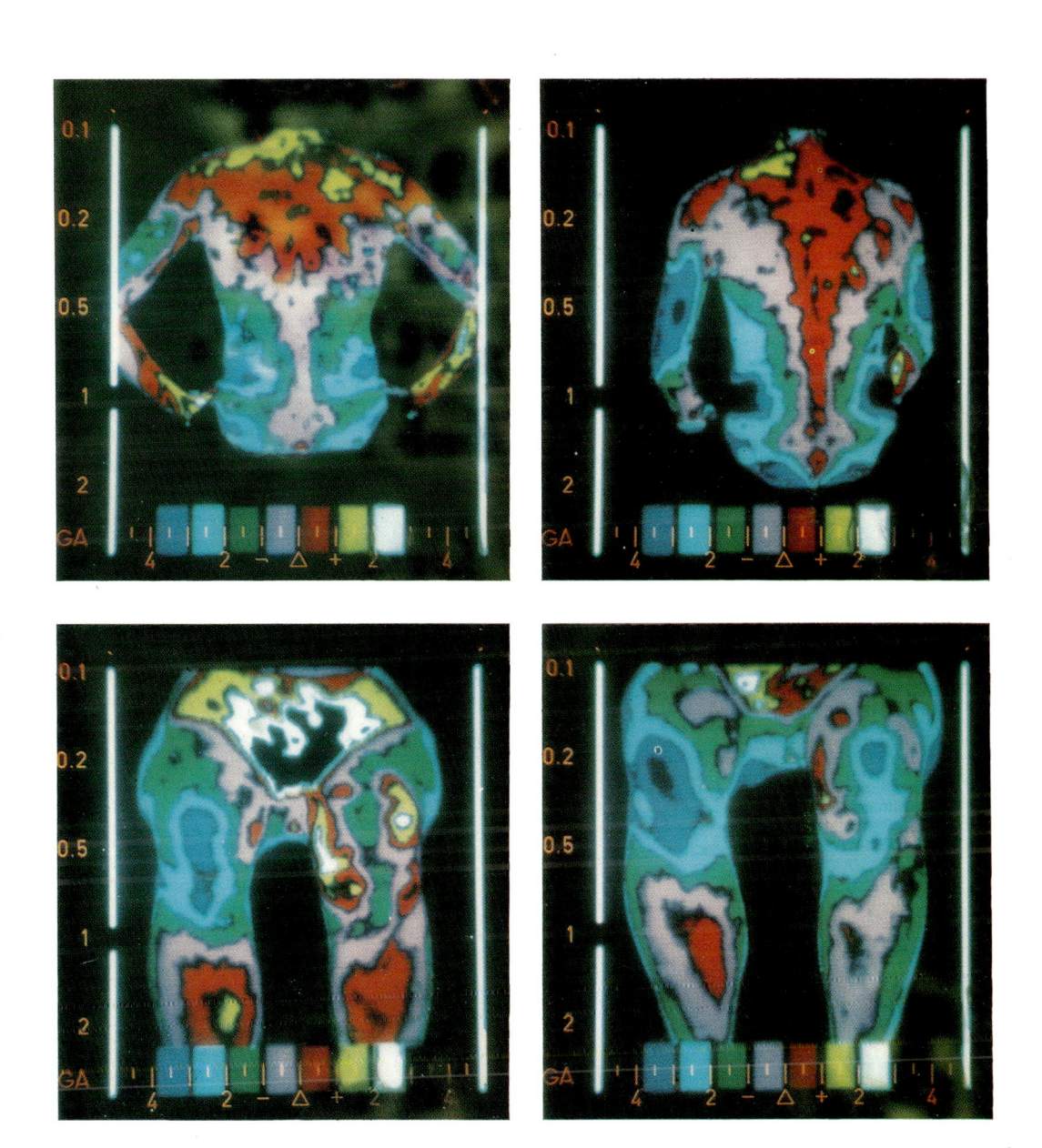

Plate 1. Thermograms of back of patient with ankylosing spondylitis (a: upper left) before diflunisal, (b: upper right) after 2 weeks' treatment.

Plate 2. Thermograms of knee of patient with ankylosing spondylitis (a: lower left) before treatment, (b: lower right) after 2 weeks' treatment with diflunisal.

"The Acute Painful Shoulder"

The shoulder joint mechanism is complex and a number of painful structures lie in close proximity. Patients with extracapsular lesions are included in this study and where possible the structure involved has been specified—supraspinatous, infraspinatous, subscapularis tendinitis or subacromial bursitis. Most of these lesions can be relieved by a local injection of hydrocortisone; the site of injection being decided by application of functional anatomy. Preliminary observations with thermography have shown that clinical improvement coincides with a fall in temperature over the involved joint.

There are a number of patients in whom local injections of corticosteroids may not be appropriate and this study has set out to compare the efficacy of diflunisal 500 mg b.i.d. to Distalgesic in patients with extracapsular lesions of less than 10 days duration.

Diflunisal has been shown to give more satisfactory pain relief than Distalgesic and thermograms have shown a fall in temperature which coincides with this improvement.

Comment

These preliminary studies have demonstrated the efficacy of diflunisal in these diverse conditions. A low incidence of side effects has been recorded. They have shown that thermography provides both an objective and sensitive way of assessing joint inflammation. It is of some importance that clinical improvement has been associated with improvement in the thermogram and has therefore demonstrated that diflunisal has an anti-inflammatory as well as an analgesic effect. Thermography has provided a useful objective non-invasive method of drug assessment in "soft-tissue rheumatism", an area of rheumatology in which objective methods of assessment are at present sadly lacking.

Acknowledgement

These pilot studies were undertaken at Addenbrookes Hospital with the collaboration of Drs Dianne Bulgen, M. de Silva, D. P. Page Thomas and Ian Shaw, and from part of a comprehensive survey of the value of thermography in non-articular rheumatism.

Summary

The assessment of disease activity in the rheumatic diseases remains a problem, as inflammation is difficult to measure in clinical practice. At the present time there is no single, ideal measurement and, therefore, it is important to use a combination of both subjective and objective methods. Thermography requires complicated equipment and strictly controlled environmental conditions, but it does seem to be able to identify the degree of reducible inflammation.

Diflunisal has been assessed in the treatment of patients with rheumatoid arthritis osteoarthritis, painful stiff shoulder and acute back strain. Thermography has been used as one of the methods of assessment.

The results confirm the efficacy of diflunisal in these conditions. In the crossover trial in rheumatoid arthritis diflunisal was at least as effective as acetylsalicylic acid (ASA). The incidence of side effects was low. Diflunisal appears to be a useful new compound for a wide variety of rheumatic conditions.

Zusammenfassung

Die Abschätzung der Krankheitstätigkeit in den rheumatischen Krankheiten bleibt ein Problem, da sich eine Entzündung in der klinischen Praxis schwer messen läßt. Gegenwärtig gibt es keine einzige ideale Messung, und daher ist es wichtig, eine Kombination sowohl subjektiver- wie auch objektiver Methoden anzuwenden. Die Thermographie erfordert komplizierte Ausrüstungen und strikt kontrollierte Umweltbedingungen, scheint jedoch nicht in der Lage zu sein, das Ausmaß einer reduzierbaren Entzündung zu identifizieren.

Diflunisal ist in der Behandlung von Patienten mit rheumaartiger Arthritis-Knochen- und Gelenkentzündung, schmerzhafter steifer Schulter und akuter Rücken, belastung abgeschätzt worden. Als eine der Beurteilungsmethoden ist die Thermographie angewandt worden.

Die Ergebnisse bestätigen die Wirksamkeit von Diflunisal unter diesen Bedingungen. In dem Austauschversuch in rheumaartiger Arthritis war Diflunisal zumindest ebenso wirksam wie Azetylsalizylsäure (ASA). Das Auftreten von Nebenwirkungen war geringfügig. Diflunisal scheint eine nützliche neue Zusammensetzung für eine Vielzahl von rheumatischen Erkrankungen zu sein.

Resumé

L'évaluation de l'activité de la maladie dans les maladies rhumatismales pose des problèmes, car l'inflammation est difficile à mesurer dans la pratique clinique. A l'heure actuelle, il n'existe pas de mesure unique idéale; il importe donc d'utiliser une combinaison de méthodes subjectives et objectives. La thermographie exige un appareillage compliqué et des conditions de milieu rigoureusement définies, mais paraît permettre la mesure du degré d'inflammation réductible.

Le diflunisal a été essayé dans le traitement des malades atteints d'arthrite rhymatismale, d'ostéoarthrite, de raideur douloureuse de l'épaule et de lumbago aigu. La thermographie a été utilisée parmi les méthodes d'évaluation.

Less résultats confirment l'efficacité du diflunisal dans ces cas. Dans l'essai à double anonymat dans les cas d'arthrite rhumastismale, le diflunisal se montre au moins aussi efficace que l'acide acétylsalicylique. Les effets secondaires sont rares. Le diflunisal est donc un composé nouveau utile envers des états rhumastismaux divers.

Sommario

La valutazione del grado di attività di malattie reumatiche rimane un problema dato che, nella pratica clinica, le infiammazioni sono di difficile misurazione. Attualmente non vi è alcun unico metodo ideale di misurazione e di conseguenza occore impiegare una combinazione di entrambi i metodi, soggettivo e oggettivo. Per la termografia occorrono apparecchiature complicate e condizioni ambientali sotto controllo, però con essa sembra che si possa determinare il grado di infiammazione riducibile.

Si è valutata l'efficacia del diflunisal con pazienti affetti da artrite reumatoide, osteoartrite, anchilosi della spalla e distorsione dorsale acuta. Si è impiegata la termografia come uno dei metodi di valutazione.

I risultati confermano l'efficacia del diflunisal con tali affezioni. Nelle prove con scambio in pazienti affetti da artrite reumatoide il diflunisal si mostrò per lo meno efficace come l'acido acetilsalicilico (AAS). L'incidenza di effetti secondari fu bassa. Dai risultati appare che il diflunisal costituisca un medicamento utile con numerose affezioni reumatiche.

Resumen

La evaluación del grado de actividad en los procesos reumáticos continúa siendo un problema, ya que es difícil medir la inflamación en la práctica clínica. Hasta el momento no hay una medida única e ideal y, por lo tanto, es importante usar ambos métodos, objetivo y subjetivo. A pesar de que la termografía requiere equipo complicado y condiciones ambientales estrictamente controladas, parece eficaz para identificar el grado de inflamación reducible.

El diflunisal se ha evaluado en el tratamiento de pacientes con artritis reumatoidea, artrosis, rigidez dolorosa en el hombro y lumbago agudo. La termografía se ha usado como uno de los métodos de evaluación.

Los resultados confirman la eficacia del diflunisal en estos casos. En los estudios cruzados de artritis reumatoidea, el diflunisal resultó al menos tan eficaz como el ácido acetilsalicílico (AAS). Hubo incidencia de efectos secundarios. El diflunisal parece ser una nueva y útil preparación para el tratamiento de gran diversidad de condiciones reumáticas.

Sumário

A avaliação da actividade da doença em afecções reumáticas continua a ser um problema, visto que a inflamação é difícil de medir na prática clínica. Presentemente não existe nenhum sistema simples e ideal de medida e, portanto, é importante que seja usada uma combinação de métodos subjectivos e objectivos. A termografia exige equipamento complicado e condições ambientes estritamente controladas, mas é um método que parece ser capaz de identificar o grau de inflamação reduzível.

O diflunisal foi objecto de estudos de avaliação no tratamento de doentes com artrite reumatóide, osteo-artrite, anquilose dolorosa do ombro e entorse costal aguda. Um dos métodos de avaliação empregados foi a termografia.

Os resultados confirmam a eficacia do diflunisal nestas afecções. Num ensaio cruzado, em artrite reumatóide, o diflunisal foi pelo menos tão eficaz como o ácido acetilsalicílico (ASA). A incidência de efeitos secundários foi baixa. O diflunisal parece ser um novo composto de utilidade para tratamento duma grande variedade de afecções reumáticas.

Clinical Reports (1)
Diflunisal Compared with Placebo in Acute Untreated Lumbago

V. JAEGEMANN

Freising, West Germany

This is a preliminary report on results obtained in a small double-blind placebo-controlled, completely randomized study with diflunisal 500 mg b.i.d. in 30 patients with acute untreated lumbago.

Methods and Patients

A diagnosis of lumbago (low back pain) with acute onset of symptoms or occurring as an acute exacerbation of chronic low back pain with bothersome low back pain and a considerable degree of functional disability were the major admission criteria. Patients who had taken a regular course of treatment with analgesics, anti-inflammatory or muscle relaxant agents were not accepted.

The patients were allocated to either placebo (5 female, 10 male) or diflunisal (10 female, 5 male) whose ages ranged between 18–58 (mean 35) in the diflunisal group and 21–46 (mean 37) in the placebo group. The duration of treatment was 7 days.

The following clinical measurements were made before therapy, and during the study on day 3 and day 7: (1) low back pain, (2) fingers to floor test, (3) postural deviation, (4) side bending, (5) functional disability, and (6) pain irradiating into the leg. A scoring system ranging from "no pain" = 0 to "severe" = 3, with moderate (2) and mild (1), was used to assess the clinical improvement.

Results

All the clinical measurements reached a statistically significant improvement in favour of diflunisal at day 3 and 7. A pronounced decrease of low back pain was obvious in

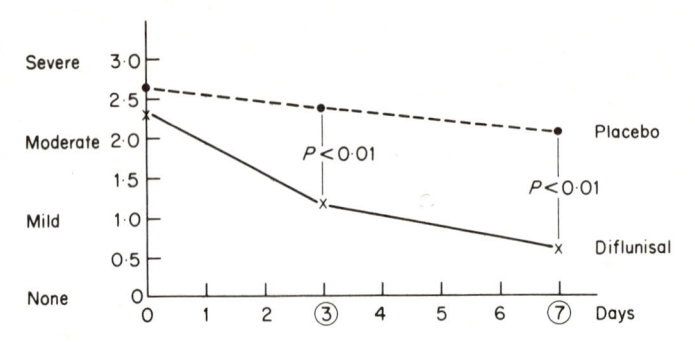

Figure 1. Assessment of severity of low back pain.

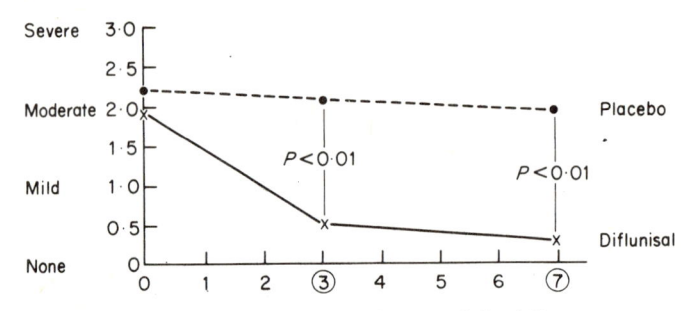

Figure 2. Improvement in functional disability.

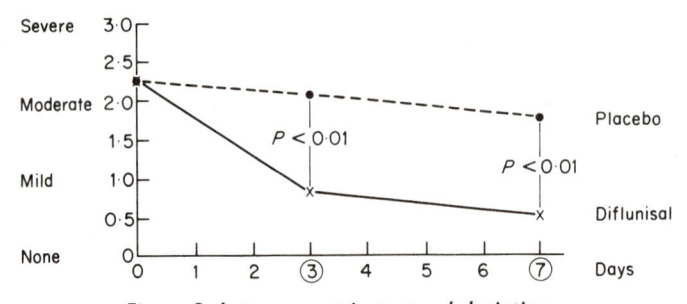

Figure 3. Improvement in postural deviation.

the diflunisal group after 3 days and at 7 days with a significance of $P<0.01$ (Fig. 1). Both functional disability (Fig. 2) and postural deviations (Fig. 3) showed clear and marked improvement in the diflunisal over placebo group, ($P<0.01$).

The fingers to floor test done on day 0, day 3 and day 7 gives a clear picture of the patient's objective improvement of mobility. This improved by 18 cm at day 3 and 22 cm at day 7 in the diflunisal group compared with 3 and 4 cm respectively on placebo.

The patients' subjective and the investigator's final evaluation of efficacy is shown in Table 1. The results indicate a statistically significant difference over the placebo group ($P<0.01$). Adverse experiences were mild in all cases; they had occurred at the beginning of the study and subsided after application of an antacid. One patient

Table 1

Patient and investigator evaluation

Evaluation	Day 3 Placebo	Day 3 Diflunisal	Day 7 Placebo	Day 7 Diflunisal
Patient:				
Excellent	0	8	0	9
Good	0	4	1	2
Fair	6	2	2	3
Poor	9	1	12	0
Investigator:				
Excellent			0	10
Good			1	2
Fair			2	1
Poor			12[a]	2[a]

[a] Includes 8 (placebo) and 1 (diflunisal) who discontinued on day 3 through lack of efficacy.

taking diflunisal had mild stomach pain and one moderate pain with nausea and vomiting. In the placebo group one patient had mild stomach pain with heartburn.

Conclusion

In this short study diflunisal has proven to be an excellent and safe therapeutic agent in the treatment of acute lumbago.

Summary

This completely randomized, double-blind study was performed to compare the efficacy and safety of diflunisal 500 mg b.i.d. to that of placebo in 30 outpatients with acute lumbago. Therapy lasted for one week. Patients were observed for various efficacy variables on days 0, 3 and 7.

Two of the 15 patients in the diflunisal group and one of the 15 in the placebo group reported mild gastrointestinal side-effects. One patient in the diflunisal group had to be withdrawn from the study because of insufficient therapeutic response, compared to eight in the placebo group.

The diflunisal group showed significant improvement in five of the six clinical parameters at both days of observation (3 and 7). Also the patient's and investigator's evaluations of efficacy were significantly in favour of diflunisal. In this study, diflunisal was shown to be an effective new analgesic in the treatment of acute lumbago.

Zusammenfassung

Diese völlig wahllose, "doppelt blinde" Studie wurde durchgeführt, um die Wirksamkeit und Sicherheit von zweimal täglich verabreichten 500 mg Diflunisal mit derjenigen von Placebo in 30 ambulanten Patienten mit akutem Hexenschuß zu vergleichen. Die Therapie dauerte eine Woche. Die Patienten wurden auf verschiedene Wirksamkeitsvariablen an den Tagen 0, 3 und 7 beobachtet.

Zwei der 15 Patienten in der Diflunisal-Gruppe und einer der 15 in der Placebo-Gruppe meldeten leichte gastrointestinale Nebenwirkungen. Ein Patient in der Diflunisal-Gruppe mußte wegen unzulänglicher therapeutischer Reaktion verglichen mit 8 in der Placebo-Gruppe von der Studie ausgeschlossen werden.

Die Diflunisal-Gruppe zeigt eine bedeutsame Verbesserung in 5 der 6 klinischen Parameter an beiden Beobachtungstagen (3 und 7). Die Auswertungen der Wirksamkeit durch den Patienten und den Untersucher sprachen ebenfalls stark zugunsten von Diflunisal. In dieser Studienarbeit wurde nachgewiesen, daß Diflunisal ein wirksames neues Analgetikum in der Behandlung von akutem Hexenschuß ist.

Resumé

Cette étude à double anonymat entièrement aléatorisée a été faire pour comparer l'efficacité et l'innocuité du diflunisal (2×500 mg par jour) à celles d'un placebo chez 30 malades ambulatoires souffrant de lumbago aigu. Le traitement durait une semaine. Les malades étaient soumis à des mesures de diverses variables d'efficacité aux jours 0, 3 et 7.

Deux des quinze malades du groupe "diflunisal" et un des quinze malades du groupe "placebo' ont signalé des effets secondaires gastro-intestinaux légers. Un des malades du groupe "diflunisal" a dû être exclu de l'étude par suite d'une réaction thérapeutique insuffisante, contre huit dans le groupe "placebo".

Le groupe "diflunisal" présentait une amélioration significative de 5 paramètres cliniques sur 6 aux jours d'observation (3 et 7). Les appréciations d'efficacité du malade et de l'investigateur étaient significativement en faveur du diflunisal. Cette étude montre que le diflunisal est un analgésique nouveau efficace dans le traitement du lumbago aigu.

Sommario

Questo studio completamente casualizzato e "double-blind" venne eseguito per confrontare l'efficacia e sicurezza del diflunisal (500 mg due volte al giorno) con quella di un placebo (sostanza innocua di controllo) in 30 pazienti esterni affetti da lombaggine acuta. La terapia ebbe la durata di una settimana. Nei giorni 0, 3 e 7 si osservò l'efficacia sui pazienti (suddivisa in vari parametri).

Due dei 15 pazienti del gruppo diflunisal e uno dei 15 del gruppo placebo dichiararono lievi effetti secondari gastro-intestinali. Per insufficienza di risposta terapeutica, si dovettero ritirare un paziente dal gruppo di diflunisal e invece 8 dal gruppo placebo.

Il gruppo diflunisal mostrò miglioramenti significativi in 5 dei 6 parametri clinici, in entrambi i giorni di osservazione (3 e 7). Pure il giudizio dei pazienti e degli indagatori circa l'efficacia fu significativamente in favore del diflunisal. In questo studio il diflunisal si mostrò essere un analgesico efficace nel trattamento della lombaggine acuta.

Resumen

Este estudio totalmente aleatorio a doble ciego se realizó para comparar la eficacia y seguridad del diflunisal en dosis de 500 mg dos veces al día en 30 pacientes externos con lumbago agudo en relación con un placebo. La terapia duró una semana. Se observaron varias variables de eficacia en los pacientes los días 0, 3 y 7.

Dos de los 15 pacientes en el grupo del diflunisal y uno de los 15 en el grupo del placebo comunicaron efectos secundarios gastrointestinales leves. Se tuvo que retirar del estudio a uno de los pacientes en el grupo del diflunisal, debido a la insuficiente respuesta terapéutica, en comparación con 8 en el grupo del placebo.

El grupo del diflunisal mostró considerable mejoría en 5 de los 6 parámetros clínicos en ambos días de observación (3 y 7). Asimismo, la evaluación de los pacientes y de los investigadores confirmaron mucho la eficacia del diflunisal. En este estudio, el diflunisal demostró ser un nuevo analgésico eficaz para el tratamiento del lumbago agudo.

Sumário

Este estudo duplamente às cegas e totalmente ao acaso foi realizado com o fim de comparar a eficácia e grau de segurança do diflunisal (500 mg duas vezes por dia) com o efeito dum placebo, em 30 doentes com lumbago agudo. A terapêutica durou uma semana. Os doentes foram examinados para observação de diversas variáveis de eficácia, nos dias 0, 3 e 7.

Dois dos 15 doentes to grupo diflunisal e um dos 15 do grupo placebo queixaram-se de ligeiros efeitos secundários gastro-intestinais. No grupo diflunisal, um doente teve de ser retirado do estudo devido a insuficiente resposta terapêutica, em comparação com 8 doentes no grupo placebo. O grupo diflunisal mostrou melhoras significativas em 5 dos 6 parâmetros clínicos, em ambos os dias de observação (3 e 7). Além disso, as avaliações de eficácia, tanto pelo doente como pelo investigador, foram significativamente em favor do diflunisal. Neste estudo, o diflunisal provou ser um novo analgésico eficaz para tratamento de lumbago agudo.

Clinical Reports (2)
Diflunisal versus Oxyphenbutazone in the Management of Pain Associated with Sprains and Strains

P. BERNETT and P. PRIMBS

Munich, West Germany

The object of this double-blind study in 40 patients with acute post-traumatic sprains and strains of the ankle or wrist, was to compare the safety and efficacy of diflunisal 375 mg b.i.d. with oxyphenbutazone 200 mg b.i.d. over a period of 5 days.

Patients and Methods

The study was completely randomized and the double-blind nature was ensured by using double-dummy medication. Practically all the patients were young sport students with a mean age of 25 years. They were examined within 60 min after injury and all had a degree of pain requiring analgesic treatment. To exclude fractures, X-rays were taken in all cases and pre-treatment standard laboratory determinations were done. Patients were excluded if they were pregnant or had aspirin hypersensitivity or any contraindication to oxyphenbutazone. Clinical assessment of response to treatment including spontaneous pain, limitation of passive movement, tenderness, swelling and limitation of active motion, was made throughout the study at days 0, 3 and 5 by two investigators. In addition, patients' evaluation of response and the investigator's evaluation of efficacy were assessed. Symptoms were rated on a 0 to 3-point scale; 0 representing none, 1=mild, 2=moderate and 3=severe.

In the diflunisal group of 20 patients, four were lost to follow-up; in the oxyphenbutazone group one patient was lost to follow-up and another was excluded from the data analysis as he had taken only half of the test drug because of an adverse reaction. A statistical analysis was performed; all variables being analysed by non-parametric tests which were run at the 5% significance level.

Diflunisal: Royal Society of Medicine International Congress and Symposium Series No. 6, published jointly by Academic Press Inc. (London) Ltd., and the Royal Society of Medicine.

Results

In the 34 patients completing the study, injuries of the ankle were predominant (29) and there were twice as many severe injuries in the diflunisal group (8/16) as in the placebo group (4/18). The sex distribution was 23 males and 11 females, the mean age was 25 years and there were no secondary diagnoses.

When looking at the results of the five clinical measurements (Figs 1 to 5) it is clear

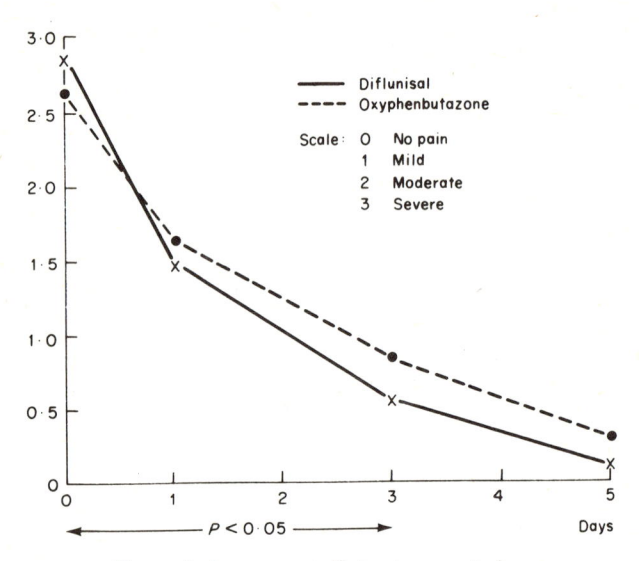

Figure 1. Assessment of spontaneous pain.

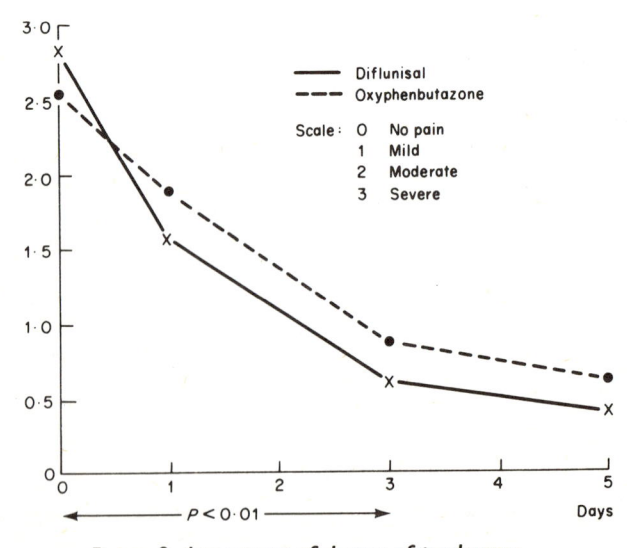

Figure 2. Assessment of degree of tenderness.

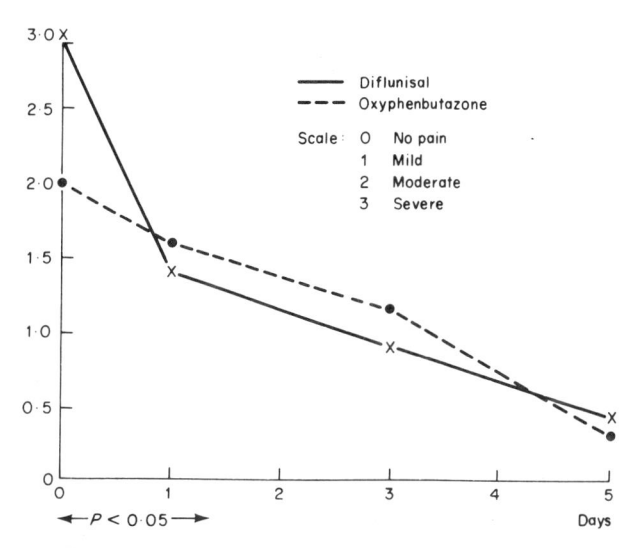

Figure 3. Improvement in limitation of active motion.

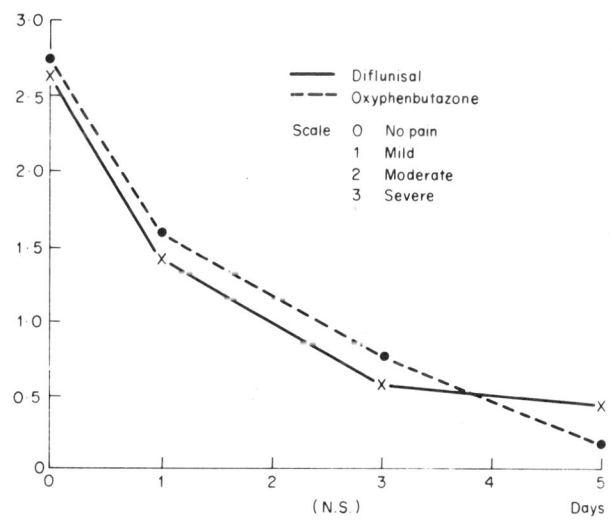

Figure 4. Improvement in limitation of passive motion.

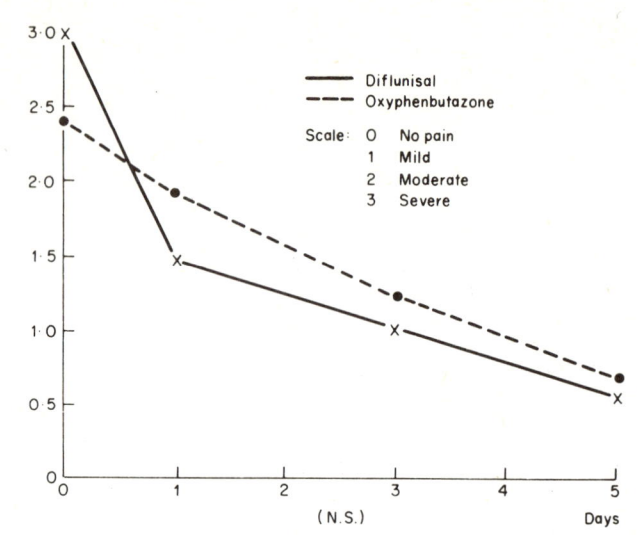

Figure 5. Assessment of reduction in swelling.

that diflunisal and oxyphenbutazone act in different ways. In the diflunisal group there was statistically a more significant improvement during the first three days of therapy and this applies specifically to spontaneous pain, tenderness and limitation of active motion.

For both compounds in relation to severity of injury in respect to the improvement in spontaneous pain, from baseline to day 3 this was statistically significant ($P<0.05$). with both treatments as did change in limitation of active motion ($P<0.01$) from baseline to day 1. There was no statistically significant difference between groups in change from baseline for limitation of passive motion or for swelling.

The distribution of patients with excellent or good response on day 1 was statistically significant in favour of diflunisal over oxyphenbutazone ($P<0.05$). The evaluation of response was assessed by the patient's opinion during and at the end of the study. There was no adverse reaction in the diflunisal group but in the oxyphenbutazone group there was one patient with mild fatigue and one patient with moderate nausea.

Conclusion

Diflunisal showed
    (1) a quicker onset of action in selected parameters,
    (2) good efficacy,
    (3) excellent tolerance.

Table 1

Patient evaluation of response

Patients' evaluation	Diflunisal	Oxyphenbutazone
Day 1: Exc/Good	10[a]	3
Fair/Poor	6	14
Day 3: Exc/Good	13	15
Fair/Poor	3	3
Day 5: Exc/Good	15	17
Fair/Poor	1	1

[a] $P<0.05$ in favour of diflunisal.

Summary

In a clinical double-blind completely randomized study of the efficacy and safety of diflunisal 375 mg b.i.d. was compared to that of oxyphenbutazone 200 mg b.i.d. in the treatment of minor sprains and strains in sports injuries; the duration of treatment being 5 days.

Forty patients (20 per group) entered the study and all were initially comparable in terms of a number of demographic and injury related variables, including signs and symptoms. The results of treatment were assessed on, spontaneous pain, tenderness, and limitation of active and passive movement. Diflunisal proved to be as effective as oxyphenbutazone in its anti-inflammatory and analgesic effect. Two patients in the oxyphenbutazone group and none in the diflunisal group reported side effects.

The overall conclusion is that, at the doses used in this study, diflunisal is better than oxyphenbutazone in the treatment of acute strains and sprains.

Zusammenfassung

In einer klinischen, "doppelt" blinden, völlig wahllosen Untersuchung wurde die Wirksamkeit und Sicherheit von zweimal täglich verabreichten 375 mg Diflunisal mit derjenigen von zweimal täglich verabreichten 200 mg Oxyphenbutazon in der Behandlung von Verstauchungen und Verrenkungen in Sportverletzungen verglichen; die Behandlungsdauer betrug 5 Tage.

Vierzig Patienten (20 je Gruppe) meldeten sich zu der Untersuchung, und alle waren anfangs hinsichtlich einer Anzahl demographischer- und verletzungsbezogener Variablen einschließlich Anzeichen und Symptomen vergleichbar. Die Ergebnisse der Behandlung wurden auf spontanem Schmerz, Empfindlichkeit und Begrenzung aktiver und passiver Bewegung beurteilt. Diflunisal erwies sich in seiner entzündungsverhindernden und analgesischen Wirkung als ebenso wirksam wie Oxyphenbutazon. Zwei Patienten in der Oxyphenbutazon-Gruppe und keiner in der Diflunisal-Gruppe meldeten Nebenwirkungen.

Die Gesamtschlußfolgerung lautet dahingehend, daß Diflunisal mit den in dieser Studie benutzten Dosen in der Behandlung von akuten Verstauchungen und Verrenkungen besser ist als Oxyphenbutazon.

Resumé

Dans une étude clinique à double anonymat entièrement aléatorisée, on compare l'efficacité et de l'innocuité du diflunisal (2×375 mg par jour) à celles de l'oxyphenbutazone (2×200 mg par jour) dans le traitement des petites foulures et élongations musculaires chez des sportifs, la durée du traitement étant de 5 jours.

Quarante malades (20 par groupe) participent à l'étude, et tous sont initialement comparables d'après un certain nombre de variables démographiques et de variables relatives aux lésions, y compris les signes et symptômes. Les résultats du traitement sont évalués aux points de vue douleur spontanée, sensibilité, et limitation des mouvements actifs et passifs. Le diflunisal se montre aussi efficace que l'oxyphenbutazone par ses effets anti-inflammatoires et analgésiques. Deux des malades du groupe "oxyphenbutazone" signalent des effets secondaires, aucun dans le groupe "diflunisal".

On en conclut qu'aux doses étudiées, le diflunisal est supérieur à l'oxyphenbutazone dans le traitement des foulures et élongations musculaires aiguës.

Sommario

In uno studio clinico completamente casualizzato e "double-blind", si sono comparate l'efficacia e sicurezza del diflunisal (375 mg due volte al giorno) con quelle dell' ossifenbutazene (200 mg due volte al giorno) nel trattamento di lievi distorsioni sportive. Durata del trattamento 5. giorni.

Fecero parte dello studio quaranta pazienti (20 per gruppo), tutti inizialmente comparabili per quanto riguarda i parametri demografici e relativi alla lesione presi in considerazione, compresi segni e sintomi. I risultati del trattamento vennero valutati basandosi su: dolorosità spontanea e al tatto; limitazione ai movimenti attivi e passivi. Il diflunisal mostrò la stessa efficacia antiflogistica e analgesica dell' ossifenbutazene. Due pazienti del gruppo ossifenbutazene e nessuno di quello diflunisal dichiararono effetti secondari.

Come conclusione generale si può affermare che, alle dosi impiegate nel presente studio, il diflunisal è migliore dell'ossifenbutazene nel trattamento di distorsioni acute.

Resumen

En un estudio clínico a doble ciego totalmente al azar, acerca de la eficacia y seguridad del diflunisal, se comparó el empleo de dosis de 375 mg dos veces diarias con otra de 200 mg, también dos veces al día, de oxifenbutazona, en el tratamiento de esguinces y desgarramientos en lesiones deportivas; la duración del tratamiento fue de 5 días.

Cuarenta pacientes (en grupos de 20) participaron en el estudio y todos eran comparables en un principio, respecto a numerosas variables demográficas y otras relacionadas con las lesiones, incluidas señales y síntomas. Se evaluaron los resultados del tratamiento en cuanto al dolor espontáneo, el dolor a la palpación y la limitación del movimiento activo y pasivo. El diflunisal demostró ser tan eficaz como la oxifenbutazona en su efecto antinflamatorio y analgésico. Dos pacientes en el grupo de la oxifenbutazona y ninguno en el del diflunisal experimentaron efectos secundarios.

La conclusión general es que el diflunisal es mejor que la oxifenbutazona, en el tratamiento de esguinces y desgarramientos agudos, en las dosis usadas en este estudio.

Sumário

Num estudo clínico, duplamente às cegas e totalmente ao acaso, a eficácia e grau de segurança do diflunisal (375 mg duas vezes por dia) foi comparada com a do oxifenbutazeno (200 mg duas vezes por dia) no tratamento de entorses ligeiras e distensões sofridas em consequência de actividades desportivas; a duração do tratamento foi de 5 dias.

Quarenta doentes (20 por grupo) participaram no estudo, e todos eles eram inicialmente comparáveis em função de certas variáveis demográficas e relacionadas com a lesão, incluindo indícios e sintomas. Os resultados do tratamento foram avaliados quanto a: dor espontânea, sensibilidade dolorosa, e limitação de movimento activo e passivo. O diflunisal provou ser tão eficaz como o oxifenbutazeno no que respeita a efeito anti-inflamatório e analgésico. Dois doentes no grupo oxifenbutazeno queixaram-se de efeitos secundários, mas no grupo diflunisal não houve quaisquer queixas deste tipo.

A conclusão global é que, às doses usadas neste estudo, o diflunisal é melhor do que o oxifenbutazeno para tratamento de entorses e distensões agudas.

Clinical Reports (3)
Diflunisal compared with ASA in Osteoarthritis

G. HOLZGARTNER

Erding, West Germany

This study forms part of multi-clinic controlled titration study in outpatients, comparing the ong-term safety and efficacy of diflunisal 500-750 mg/day with acetylsalicylic acid (ASA), 2-3 g/day. The first 12 weeks were double-blind and the patients were randomly assigned to the study; thereafter, the study was open.

Patients and Methods

Patients were admitted to the study who had a confirmed diagnosis of osteoarthritis of the hip or knee with local pain relieved by rest, limitation of movement, positive X-ray findings, inactivity stiffness and night pain. The major exclusion criteria were ASA hypersensitivity, systemic steroid therapy, other joint diseases and abnormal laboratory values. At the start of the study the diflunisal group had five female and seven male patients; in the ASA group there were seven females and three male patients. As it progressed, quite a few dropped out for various reasons but out of the 12 patients who had entered the diflunisal part, four remained with this therapy and are presently in week 133. Only two patients of the ASA group continued up to week 48. The ages ranged from 22 to 66 with a mean of 54 in the diflunisal group and 47 to 70 with a mean of 61 in the ASA group. The major joint of involvement in the diflunisal group was the hip in seven patients and the knee in five; in the ASA group the figures were five and five.

Clinical improvement was assessed twice weekly for the first two weeks and once a month up to week 24. Thereafter assessment was made every two months and subsequently every three months. The measurements carried cut are listed in Table 1. Weight, blood pressure and laboratory values were also controlled at these visits.

Diflunisal: Royal Society of Medicine International Congress and Symposium Series No. 6, published jointly by Academic Press Inc. (London) Ltd., and the Royal Society of Medicine.

Table 1

Clinical assessment measurements

Weight bearing pain
Inactivity stiffness (min)
Night pain
Choice of activity giving most trouble
(a) getting out of bed
(b) getting up from a chair
(c) Walking a stated distance
(d) Climbing stairs
Knee flexion (degrees)
Intermalleolar distance

Results

Weight bearing pain (Fig. 1)

Diflunisal achieved a statistical significance ($P<0.01$) over ASA during the entire study period. There were significantly more patients with severe pre-treatment weight bearing pain in the diflunisal group.

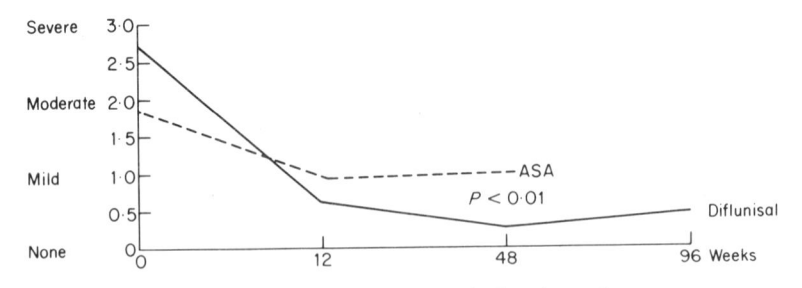

Figure 1. Assessment of weight bearing pain.

Night pain (Fig. 2)

There was a statistical significance ($P<0.01$) for diflunisal, although in this case the initial intensity of night pain was somewhat more severe in the ASA group.

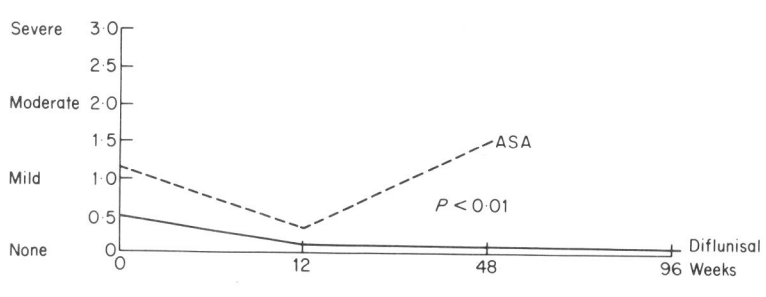

Figure 2. Assessment of night pain.

Adverse experiences

In the diflunisal group adverse experiences were observed in two patients with mild and three with moderate gastrointestinal symptoms, two patients with moderate and one severe dry muccus membranes, and one man reported painful nipples. These nine side effects involved seven patients over 96 weeks. In the ASA group there were two patients with mild, two with moderate and three with severe gastrointestinal complaints. Two patients had severe CNS symptoms (nausea and dizziness), one patient had a mild exanthema, and there was one patient with mild and two with moderate symptoms in the respiratory system. Two patients had dry mucous membranes of mild degree. In this group, these 15 side effects involved six patients over 48 weeks.

Withdrawal from treatment

In the diflunisal group a total of eight of the initial 12 dropped out but the remaining four are still progressing after 133 weeks. Those dropping out were two because of adverse clinical experience, one because of inefficacy, two were lost to follow-up and three dropped out for personal reasons, such as change of residence etc.

In the ASA group all 10 stopped at week 48, six because of adverse clinical experience, two because of inefficacy, one was lost to follow-up and one underwent surgery.

So far no adverse laboratory values have been observed and there has been no significant difference between the investigator's and the patients' evaluation of efficacy, both favouring diflunisal over ASA.

Conclusion

Diflunisal has proven to be an effective and safe medication in the long-term treatment of osteoarthritis of the hip or knee over a period of 96 and 133 weeks respectively.

Summary

A double-blind completely randomized, multi-centred, controlled titration study in outpatients comparing the safety and efficacy of diflunisal (500–750 mg/day) against acetylsalicyclic acid (2·0–3·0 g/day) was carried out over a period of 12 weeks. Twelve patients were entered into the diflunisal and 10 into the ASA group with a diagnosis of either osteoarthritis of the hip or knee.

After week 12, the study was open and patients received the medication according to the maintenance dose established. During the course of this long-term study which has now extended to 133 weeks, eight patients in the ASA group dropped our—mostly because of adverse reactions—by the end of week 12. The last two patients dropped out at weeks 32 and 48, respectively. In the diflunisal group, all patients completed week 12, seven patients completed week 48 (two patients dropped out because of adverse experience, three patients were lost to follow-up), and four patients are presently ongoing. Side effects in the ASA as well as in the diflunisal group were of gastrointestinal origin.

Diflunisal proved to be effective and safe in long-term treatment of osteoarthritis of the hip or knee.

Zusammenfassung

Es wurde eine doppelt blinde, völlig wahllose, mehrfachzentrierte, kontrollierte Titrationsuntersuchung in ambulanten Patienten zum Vergleich der Sicherheit und Wirksamkeit von Diflunisal (500–750 mg/Tag) mit Azetylsalizylsäure (2,0–3,0 g/Tag) über einen Zeitraum von 12 Wochen durchgeführt. Zwölf Patienten wurden der Diflunisal-Gruppe und 10 der ASA-Gruppe zugeteilt, und zwar mit einer Diagnose von Osteoarthritis entweder der Hüfte oder des Knies.

Nach der Woche 12 war die Studie offen, und die Patienten erhielten die Medikation in der festgesetzten Dauerdosis. Im Verlaufe dieser langfristigen Studie, die sich nunmehr auf 133 Wochen erstreckt hat, waren 8 Patienten der ASA-Gruppe bis zum Ende der Woche 12 hauptsächlich wegen widriger Reaktionen ausgefallen. In den Wochen 32 bzs. 48 fielen die letzten beiden Patienten aus. In der Diflunisal-Gruppe beendeten alle Patienten Woche 12, 7 Patienten beendeten Woche 48 (2 Patienten fielen wegen widriger Erfahrungen aus, 3 Patienten konnten nicht weiterverfolgt werden), und 4 Patienten machen zurzeit weiter. Nebenwirkungen in der SAS- sowie in der Diflunisal-Gruppe waren gastrointestinalen Ursprungs.

Diflunisal erwies sich in der langfristigen Behandlung von Osteoarthritis der Hüfte oder des Knies als wirksam und sicher.

Résumé

Une étude de dosage contrôlée pluricentrique à double anonymat entièrement aléatorisée, destinée à comparer l'innocuité et l'efficacité du diflunisal (500–750 mg/jour) et de l'acide acétylsalicylique (2,0–3,0 g/jour), a été effectuée sur une période de 12 semaines. Douze malades faisaient partie du groupe "diflunisal" et deux du groupe "acide acétylsalicylique", avec un diagnostic d'ostéarthrite de la hanche ou du genou.

Après la 12e semaine, les malades recevaient une médication conforme à la posologie d'entretien établie. Pendant cette étude à long terme, qui a déjà duré 133 semaines, huit malades du groupe "acide acétylsalicylique" se sont retirés à la fin de la 12e semaine, principalement par suite de réactions défavorables. Les deux derniers malades se sont retirés au bout de 32 et 48 semaines respectivement. Dans le groupe "diflunisal", tous les malades ont tenu 12 semaines; 7 malades ont tenu 48 semaines (deux malades se sont retirés par suite de résultats défavorables, trois ont été perdus de vue), et six malades poursuivent l'expérience. Les effets secondaires dans les deux groupes étaient de nature gastro-intestinale.

Le diflunisal se montre efficace et sans danger dans le traitement à long terme de l'ostéoarthrite de la hanche ou du genou.

Sommario

Per un periodo di dodici settimane si eseguì uno studio di titolazione controllata completamente casualizzato "double-blind", pluricentrato, su pazienti esterni per mettere a raffronto la sicurezza ed efficacia del diflunisal (500–750 mg/giorno) con quella dell'acido acetilsalicilico (2,0–3,0 g/giorno). Dodici pazienti facevano parte del gruppo diflunisal e 10 del gruppo AAS, tutti con diagnosi di osteoartrite dell'anca oppure del ginocchio.

Dopo 12 settimane si aprì lo studio e si somministrò ai pazienti quantità di medicinale secondo la dose di mantenimento stabilitasi. Durante il corso di questo studio a lungo termine che ora ha raggiunto 133 settimane, entro la fine della settimana 12 dal gruppo AAS si ritirarono 8 pazienti, per lo piú per via di reazoini avverse; i due ultimi pazienti si ritirarono rispettivamente alla settimana 32 e settimana 48. Nel gruppo diflunisal, tutti i pazienti completarono la settimana 12, 7 pazienti completarono la settimana 48 (2 pazienti si ritirarono per via di effetti avversi, 3 pazienti andarono perduti nell'osservazione a distanza), e 4 pazienti sono ancora in corso. Sia nel gruppo AAS che diflunisal, gli effetti secondari furono di origine gastrointestinale.

Il diflunisal si mostrò efficace e sicuro nel trattamento a lungo termine dell'osteoartrite dell'anca o del ginocchio.

Resumen

Se realizó una investigación a doble ciego, totalmente aleatoria, en varios centros, por un periodo de 12 semanas, comparando la seguridad y eficacia del diflunisal (500–750 mg al día) con la del ácido acetilsalicílico (2,0 a 3,0 g/día) por medio de estudios de dosificación controlada. Se colocaron 12 pacientes en el grupo del diflunisal y 10 en el ácido acetilsalicílico, con diagnosis de artrosis de cadera o rodilla.

Después de la duodécima semana, se inició el estudio y los pacientes recibieron las medicinas de acuerdo con la dosis de mantenimiento estableciad. Durante este estudio a largo plazo, que ahora ha alcanzado la decimotercera semana, 8 pacientes tratados con ácido acetilsalicílico abandonaron el estudio al final de la duodécima semana, debido principalmente a las reacciones adversas. Los dos últimos pacientes abandonaron la investigación en las semanas número 32 y 48, respectivamente. En el grupo del diflunisal todos los pacientes llegaron a la duodécima semana, 7 pacientes llegaron a la semana 48 (2 pacientes abandonaron debido a reacciones adversas y 3 pacientes no se localizaron en los controles clínicos posteriores) y 4 pacientes siguen todavía en el estudio. Los efectos secundarios en el grupo de AAS y, asimismo, del diflunisal fueron de origen gastrointestinal.

El diflunisal demostró ser eficaz y seguro en el tratamiento a largo plazo de la artrosis de cadera o de rodilla.

Sumário

Um estudo de titulação controlada foi efectuado durante um período de 12 semanas, numa base duplamente às cegas e totalmente ao acaso, em doentes externos de vários centros, destinado a comparar a eficácia e grau de segurança do diflunisal (500–750 mg/dia) com a do ácido acetilsalicílico (2,0–3,0 g/dia). O grupo diflunisal era formado por 12 doentes e o grupo ASA por 10 doentes, todos com diagnóstico de osteo-artrite da anca ou do joelho.

Ao fim das 12 semanas, o estudo foi aberto e os doentes continuaram a ser medicados em conformidade com a dose de manutenção estabelecida. Durante este estudo a longo-prazo, cuja duração se estende agora a 133 semanas, 8 doentes no grupo ASA abandonaram o tratamento—principalmente devido a reacções adversas—ao fim da 12ª semana. Os dois doentes restantes, abandonaram à 32^a e 48ª semanas, respectivamente. No grupo diflunisal, todos os doentes completaram a 12ª semana, 7 doentes completaram a 48ª semana (2 doentes abandonaram devido a efeitos adversos e 3 doentes deixaram de comparecer e, portanto, não puderam ser seguidos). e finalmente 4 doentes estão prosseguindo com o tratamento ainda presentemente, Os efeitos secundários tanto no grupo ASA como no grupo diflunisal foram de origem gastro-intestinal.

O diflunisal provou ser eficaz e de segurança no tratamento a longo-prazo de osteo-artrite da anca ou do joelho.

Dr. J. E. Dippy (Swindon UK) also presented some data on a double-blind 8 week trial of aspirin (4 g/day) versus diflunisal (1 g/day) in rheumatoid arthritis.

Clinicians' and patients' subjective assessments coincided giving three successes and four failures of aspirin and seven successes and one failure on diflunisal. Changes in the parameters: day pain score, night pain score, morning stiffness, Ritchie score and grip strength all favoured diflunisal (Table 2).

Table 2

Diflunisal versus aspirin in rheumatoid arthritis mean changes (15 patients)

	Aspirin	Diflunisal
Day pain score	− 0·6	− 1·4
Night pain score	− 1·0	− 1·9
Morning stiffness (mins)	+12·1	−100·0
Ritchie score	− 7·0	− 18·4
Grip strength (mmHg)	+25·7	+115·6

The number of patients with side-effects was four for aspirin and five for diflunisal but patients on aspirin had to be withdrawn an account of inefficacy. No patient on diflunisal had epigastric discomfort, tinnitus or deafness.

A Comparative Study of Diflunisal and a Combination of Dextropropoxyphene/Paracetamol in Sprains and Strains

A. JAFFE

Bournemouth, England

Patients and Methods

Fifty-two patients of both sexes, aged 16 to 62, took part in this 3-day study and only one failed to complete the course of treatment. They were suffering from moderate to severe pain following a simple sprain or strain of a wrist or ankle which had occurred within the previous 24 h. The patients were randomly allocated to one of two treatment groups, receiving diflunisal (500 mg b.i.d.) or 2 tablets of a fixed combination of dextropropoxyphene 32·5 mg and paracetamol 325 mg t.i.d. A double-dummy administration schedule was used and each group contained 26 patients, the groups being comparable in age, sex, site and severity of injury.

In the diflunisal group, 16 patients had ankle involvement and 10 wrist involvement; the dextropropoxyphene/paracetamol group had 17 and 8 respectively. There was no difference in response between the two sites in either group, so the data were combined.

Results

Comparability

Table 1 shows the severity of injury on entry to the study; the large majority being moderate.

Table 1

Group	Mild	Moderate	Severe	Total
Diflunisal	4	18	4	26
Dextropropoxyphene/paracetamol	2	21	2	25

Diflunisal: Royal Society of Medicine International Congress and Symposium Series No. 6, published jointly by Academic Press Inc. (London) Ltd., and the Royal Society of Medicine.

Five patients in the diflunisal group and eight in the dextropropoxyphene/paracetamol group had radiographs taken and no abnormalities were seen.

In terms of sex, age, site of injury, severity of lesion and delay before treatment, there was an excellent balance between the two groups.

Side effects

One patient on diflunisal complained of a headache a few hours after the first dose but this may not have been drug induced, while one patient on dextropropoxyphene/paracetamol complained about the quantity of tablets and found them difficult to take and one refused to continue the study so was omitted from the analysis. Another patient took the tablets for 24 h, then defaulted but these 24 h results have been included.

Analgesic responses (Tables 2 and 3)

The differences in scores at the first visit and after one and three days' treatment, were recorded. None became worse during the study but, for different reasons, the responses of some patients were not available on days 1 and 3.

Table 2

Spontaneous pain and pain bearing

No. grades improvement after 1 day					Group	No. grades improvement after 3 days				
0	1	2	3	N/A		0	1	2	3	N/A
17	7	1	0	1	Diflunisal	7	14	4	1	0
11	14	0	0	0	Dextropropoxyphene/ paracetamol	2	14	8	0	1

0. poor; 1. fair; 2. good; 3. excellent.

Table 3

Weight-bearing pain

Improvement after 1 day					Group	Improvement after 3 days				
0	1	2	3	N/A		0	1	2	3	N/A
10	13	2	0	1	Diflunisal	6	14	6	0	0
13	11	1	0	0	Dextropropoxyphene/ paracetamol	5	12	7	0	1

0. poor; 1. fair; 2. good; 3. excellent.

Patient and clinical evaluations (Tables 4 and 5)

Table 4

Patients' evaluation

	Day 1				Group	Day 3				
0	1	2	3	N/A		0	1	2	3	N/A
3	12	6	3	2	Diflunisal	2	4	14	5	1
2	12	9	0	2	Dextropropoxyphene/paracetamol	0	8	13	1	3

0. poor; 1. fair; 2. good; 3. excellent.

Table 5

Clinical evaluation (at day 3)

0	1	2	3	N/A	Group
2	8	15	1	0	Diflunisal
0	6	17	1	1[a]	Dextropropoxyphene/paracetamol

0. poor; 1. fair; 2. good; 3. excellent.
[a] One patient defaulted after 24 h so was not clinically assessed at 3 days.

Discussion

Previous studies have illustrated the difficulties in evaluating analgesics in the short-term treatment of self-limiting pain. This study was undertaken as a preliminary to a larger one to define those clinical parameters most likely to show variation between the different treatments. Patients were treated with two tablets of diflunisal b.i.d. or dextropropoxyphene/paracetamol t.i.d. and both treatments were equally effective in the chosen parameters at 24 h and at 3 days. Dextropropoxyphene/paracetamol is probably the most commonly prescribed drug for this type of injury although it has recently been criticised because of its tendency to produce respiratory depression and addiction.

In a further study night pain will also be evaluated because the crucial factor of the long half-life of diflunisal indicates a different and more favourable clinical response from that of shorter acting analgesics. Also diflunisal may well have an anti-inflammatory effect on the inflammation accompanying trauma.

Appendix

In a separate randomized double-blind study comparing the efficacy and tolerance of diflunisal 500 mg b.i.d. with placebo for one week in non-skeletal low back pain data were analysed from 74 patients, 38 on diflunisal and 36 on placebo. In all parameters, including pain, posture, function, etc, at both day 3 and day 7, diflunisal was better than placebo, often markedly so. No side-effects were reported for placebo but three out of 38 patients on diflunisal reported "a muzzy head".

The marked improvement in posture between days 3 and 7 for the diflunisal group and improvement in all other symptoms, suggest the advisability of a slightly longer dosage period than 7 days (say 10 days) to achieve the optimum results. Meanwhile, it is clear that diflunisal is an effective and safe treatment for non-skeletal low back pain.

Acknowledgement

This work was carried out in Great Britain by General Practitioners of the Wessex Clinical Trials Organization.

Summary

In a multi-centred general practitioner trial in Great Britain, 52 patients suffering from moderate to severe pain following a strain or sprain of wrist or ankle joint within the preceding 24 h were treated on a double-blind basis with either diflunisal 500 mg b.i.d. (two tablets twice a day), a fixed combination of dextropropoxyphene 32·5 mg, and paracetamol (acetaminophen) 325 mg t.i.d., (two tablets t.i.d.). The response of pain to treatment in both groups was assessed by patient and clinician after 1 day and after 3 days. Both treatments were equally effective in the chosen parameters. Side-effects were minimal.

A further study incorporating additional parameters e.g., the evaluation of night pain response, has begun. Results so far indicate that diflunisal is an effective, well-tolerated and practical analgesic for use in general practice.

Zusammenfassung

In einem in mehreren Zentren von praktischen Ärzten in Großbritannien durchgeführten Versuch wurden 52 an mäßigem bis starkem Schmerz nach einer Zerrung oder Verstauchung des Hand- oder Sprunggelenks innerhalb der vorhergehenden 24 Stunden leidende Patienten auf einer doppelt blinden Basis mit entweder Diflunisal, 500 mg zweimal täglich (zwei Tabletten zweimal täglich) einer festen Kombination von Dextropropoxyphen, 32,5 mg, und Paracematol (Acetaminophen), 325 mg, zwei Tabletten dreimal täglich, behandelt. Die Reaktion des Schmerzes auf die Behandlung in beiden Gruppen wurde durch den Patienten und Kliniker nach einem Tag und nach drei Tagen abgeschätzt. Beide Behandlungen waren in den gewählten Parametern gleich wirksam. Nebenwirkungen waren minimal.

Eine weitere Studie mit zusätzlichen Parametern, z.B. die Auswertung der Nachtschmerzreaktion, hat begonnen. Die bisher erhaltenen Ergebnisse deuten an, daß Diflunisal ein wirksames, gut verträgliches und praktisches Analgetikum für Gebrauch in der allgemeinen Praxis ist.

Resumé

Dans un essai pluricentrique fait par des généralistes en Grande-Bretagne, 52 malades souffrant de douleurs modérées à violentes à la suite d'une foulure ou d'un étirement de l'articulation du poignet ou de la cheville dans les 24 heures précédentes sont traités à double anonymat par le diflunisal (2 comprimés de 500 mg par jour) ou par une combinaison de 32,5 mg de dextropropoxyphène et 325 mg de paracétamol (acétaminophène) (deux comprimés trois fois par jour). La réaction de la douleur au traitement dans les deux groupes est évaluée par le malade et par le clinicien après un jour et après trois jours. Les deux traitements sont également efficaces selon les paramètres choisis. Les effets secondaires sont minimes.

Une autre étude portant sur des paramètres complémentaires (réaction de la douleur nocturne par exemple) a été commencée. Les résultats obtenus jusqu'ici indiquent que le diflunisal est un analgésique efficace, bien toléré et pratique pour l'emploi par les généralistes.

Sommario

In una prova in un ambulatorio generale in Gran Bretagna, a 52 pazienti affetti da dolori da lievi ad acuti in seguito a distorsione di polso o caviglia entro le precedenti 24 ore si somministrarono, col metodo "double-blind", due volte al giorno 500 mg (due compresse) di diflunisal oppure, tre volte al giorno, una combinazione fissa di 32,5 mg (una compressa) di destropropossifene e 32,5 mg (una compressa) di paracetamolo (acetaminofene). In entrambi i gruppi gli effetti analgesici al trattamento vennero valutati sia dal paziente che dal medico curante dopo un giorno e tre giorni. Entrambi i trattamenti hanno rivelato la medesima efficacia per quanto riguarda i parametri prescelti. Gli effetti secondari furono minimi.

E' incominciato un ulteriore studio al quale sono stati aggiunti ulteriori parametri, come per esempio la valutazione dell'effetto analgesico contro i dolori notturni. I risultati finora ottenuti indicano che il diflunisal costituisce un'analgesico efficace, pratico e ben tollerato per impiego in studi o ambulatori di medicina generale.

Resumen

En un estudio de múltiples centros con médicos de cabecera en Gran Bretaña, se trataron a doble ciego 52 pacientes con dolor moderado a intenso de un esguince o desgarramiento en la articulación de la muñeca o del tobillo en las 24 horas previas, ya sea con 500 mg de diflunisal dos veces al día (dos comprimidos dos veces diarias), una combinación fija de dextropropoxifeno 32,5 mg y paracetamol (acetaminofen) 325 mg, dos comprimidos tres veces al día. Se evaluó en ambos grupos la respuesta del dolor al tratamiento por el informe del paciente y del médico clínico, transcurrido un día y tres días. Ambos tratamientos demostraron ser igualmente eficaces respecto a los parámetros escogidos. Hubo una incidencia mínima de efectos secundarios.

Se ha comenzado un nuevo estudio que incorpora parámetros adicionales; por ejemplo la evaluación de la repuesta al dolor nocturno. Hasta el momento, los resultados indican que el diflunisal es un analgésico eficaz bien tolerado y conveniente para uso en medicina general.

Sumário

Num ensaio em vários centros de clínica geral na Grã-Bretanha, 52 doentes sofrendo de dor moderada a severa, em seguida a distensão ou entorse da articulação do pulso ou tornoselo ocorrida durante as 24 horas precedentes, foram tratados numa base duplamente às cegas quer com 500 mg b.i.d. de diflunisal (dois comprimidos duas vezes por dia), quer com uma combinação fixa de 32,5 mg de dextropropoxifeno e 325 mg de paracetamol (acetaminofen) (dois comprimidos três vezes por dia). A resposta da dor ao tratamento, em ambos os grupos, foi avaliada pelo doente e pelo médico após um dia e após três dias. Ambos os tratamentos foram igualmente eficazes no que respeita aos parâmetros escolhidos. Os efeitos secundários foram mínimos.

Um novo estudo incorporando parâmetros adicionais, tais como a avaliação da resposta de dor nocturna, já foi iniciado. Os resultados até aqui, indicam que o diflunisal é um analgésico eficaz, bem tolerado e de uso prático, para aplicação em clínica geral.

A Comparative Clinical Trial of Diflunisal and Glafenine in the Control of Pain in Osteoarthritis

A. AXLER

*Department of Orthopaedic Surgery,
St. Clara Hospital, Rotterdam, Netherlands*

Diflunisal is a new analgesic agent, a carboxylic acid derivative, with a potency 2-16 times that of ASA in various animal models. Despite this greater potency, diflunisal produced less gastrointestinal irritation in animal and human studies (De Schepper et al., 1975).

Single-dose studies in humans have shown that diflunisal achieves peak plasma concentrations in 2-3 h. The initial plasma half-life of diflunisal appeared to be 10-12 h for the 500 mg dose (versus 2-3 h for ASA) (Steelman et al., 1975).

The purpose of this study was to compare the efficacy and safety of diflunisal with glafenine in patients with osteoarthritis of hip and/or knee.

Table 1

Demographic and diagnostic characteristics

	Diflusinal		Glafenine
15 patients:	9 females 6 males	15 patients:	10 females 5 males
mean		mean	
age	: 55·8 years	age	: 58·7 years
body weight	: 77·0 kg	body weight	: 75·7 kg
duration of oa	: 4·0 years	duration of oa	: 3·4 years
joint knee	: 7 patients	joint knee	: 5 patients
hip	: 8 patients	hip	: 10 patients

Diflunisal: Royal Society of Medicine International Congress and Symposium Series No. 6, published jointly by Academic Press Inc. (London) Ltd., and the Royal Society of Medicine.

Materials and Methods

Patient selection

Thirty ambulatory patients, 19 females and 11 males, age between 21 and 70 years with a definite diagnosis of osteoarthritis of hip and/or knee were selected. The demographic and diagnostic characteristics are listed in Table 1; no statistically significant differences were found between the treatment groups. Patients in any of the following categories were excluded from the study: evidence of the severe consolidated forms of the disease, pregnancy or a practical possibility of pregnancy, nursing mothers, hypersensitivity to salicylates or glafenine, current treatment with systemic corticosteroids or anti-coagulants, active peptic ulcer or g.i. haemorrhage, significant kidney or liver disease, haemopoietic disorders.

Concomitant use of antacids, analgesics, anti-inflammatories or local injection therapies were not permitted during the trial. Physiotherapy begun prior to the study could continue but such therapy was not to be initiated during the trial.

Table 2

Clinical and laboratory measurements

	week −1	0	2	4	8
weight-bearing pain	x	x	x	x	x
reduction functional activity	x	x	x	x	x
inactivity stiffness	x	x	x	x	x
night pain	x	x	x	x	x
patients' assessment of therapy			x	x	x
investigator's assessment of therapy			x	x	x
laboratory tests	x				x

Procedure

During the initial visit, patients were assessed by the investigator with regard to the admission criteria. Patients who were provisionally selected for the study stopped any current drug therapy for osteoarthritis and started a placebo wash-out period (one tablet t.i.d.).

Patients were to return after one week on placebo or sooner if their condition worsened. At the end of the wash-out period, patients who still satisfied the admission criteria and who complained of weight-bearing pain and of a reduction in a specific functional activity, were randomly allocated to either the diflunisal or the glafenine group.

Patients were to remain on their assigned test medication for 8 weeks: a 4-week double-blind and a 4-week open label treatment period. During the first 4 weeks of treatment, patients in the diflunisal group received one tablet of diflunisal 250 mg b.i.d. and patients in the glafenine group received one tablet of glafenine 200 mg t.i.d. Due to the different dosage forms and treatment regimens, a double-dummy technique of dose administration was used to maintain the double-blind nature of the study.

After 4 weeks of double-blind therapy, the treatment code was broken. Patients with a satisfactory response to their treatment continued with the same dosage for another 4 weeks. Patients who did not respond satisfactorily increased dosage to diflunisal 750 mg daily or to glafenine 800 mg daily. Diflunisal was given in one dose of 250 mg and one dose of 500 mg with the higher dose taken in the morning or evening corresponding to complaints being more severe during the day or night. Glafenine was given in 200 mg doses q.i.d.

The different parameters and the times of evaluation are shown in Table 2. Except for the inactivity stiffness measured in minutes, all clinical parameters were rated on a 0–3 point scale:

Pain score: 0 = none   Score for assessment of therapy: 0 = none/poor
           1 = mild   1 = fair
           2 = moderate   2 = good
           3 = severe   3 = excellent

The following laboratory data were determined: haemoglobin, WBC with differentiation, serum creatinine, total bilirubin, SGOT, and alkaline phosphatase.

Analysis

For all parameters, changes within the treatment groups were assessed by the Wilcoxon signed rank test. For age, weight, duration, weight-bearing pain, difficulty with a functional activity, night pain and inactivity stiffness, differences between treatment groups were assessed by the Kruskal-Wallis test. For the remaining parameters differences between treatment groups were assessed by a Rank-sum test for $2 \times N$ ordered contingency tables (Klotz, 1966), or by Fisher's exact test for 2×2 tables.

Results

Twenty-nine out of 30 patients completed the study. One patient was dropped out after 10 days due to an adverse reaction on diflunisal. At week 4, one patient switched to diflunisal 750 mg daily (the higher dose in the morning) and 14 patients to glafenine 200 mg q.i.d. (Fig. 1). Despite the random allocation, patients in the diflunisal group

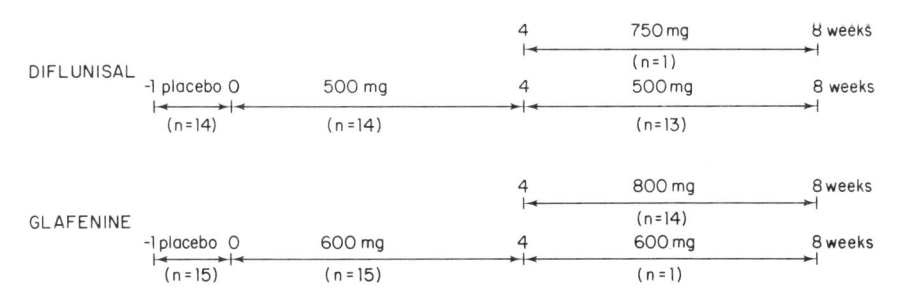

Figure 1. Study design.

exhibited more severe ratings of the parameters at baseline than did patients in the glafenine group, significantly so for weight-bearing pain ($P<0.05$) and inactivity stiffness ($P<0.05$).

The mean scores of the test drugs in weight-bearing pain, reduction in a specific functional activity, night pain and inactivity stiffness are shown in Figs 2–5. Patients in both groups responded well to their respective treatment.

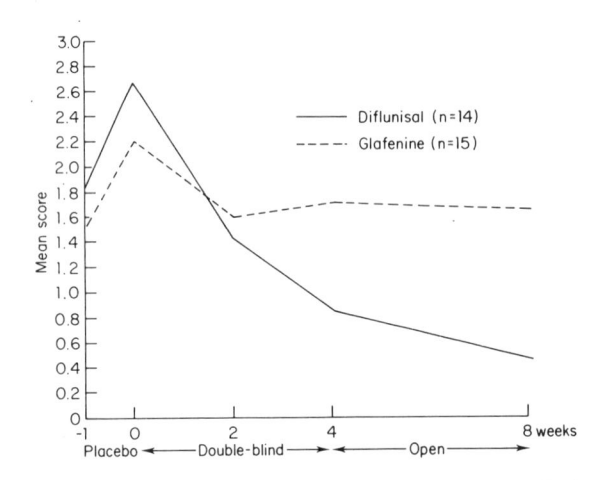

Figure 2. Comparative effect of diflunisal and glafenine on weight-bearing pain.

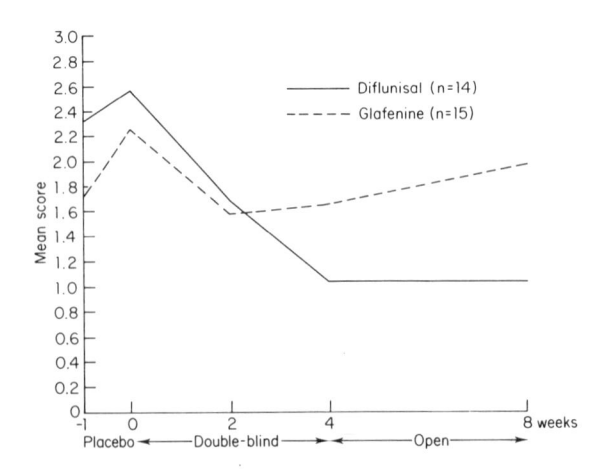

Figure 3. Comparative effect of diflunisal and glafenine on a specific functional activity.

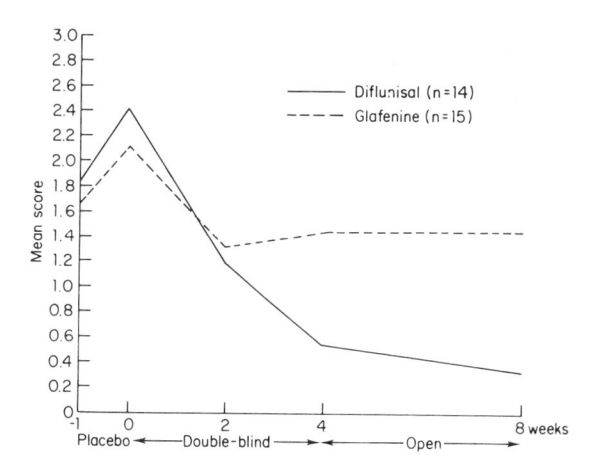

Figure 4. Comparative effect of diflunisal and glafenine on night pain.

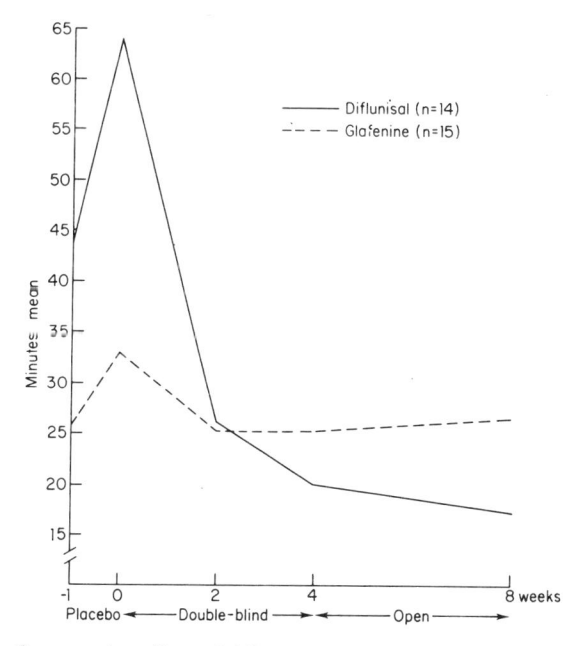

Figure 5. Comparative effect of diflunisal and glafenine on inactivity stiffness.

At weeks 4 and 8 improvement with regard to each parameter was significantly greater for the diflunisal group than for the glafenine group ($P<0.01$ in all cases).

Although at week 2 improvement with regard to each parameter was consistently greater for the diflunisal group than for the glafenine group, the difference achieved significance only for weight-bearing pain and inactivity stiffness ($P<0.01$).

At week 2, 4, and 8, the treatment groups differed significantly with regard to both the patients' and investigator's assessments of therapy. In all cases, the differences indicated a preference of the patient and the investigator to diflunisal over glafenine ($P<0.01$, except for patients' assessment week 2 $P<0.05$).

Adverse Reactions

One patient on diflunisal discontinued therapy after 10 days due to a moderate exanthema. This exanthema disappeared after a few days without treatment. In the laboratory analyses, no abnormalities were found due to the test medications.

Conclusion

The results of this study indicate that diflunisal is superior to glafenine in the treatment of osteoarthritis of hip and/or knee. Another advantage of diflunisal over glafenine is its b.i.d. dosage schedule.

References

De Schepper, P. J., Tjandramaga, T. B., Verhaest, L. and Steelman, S. L. (1975). Comparative fecal blood loss studies with a new analgesic (MK-647) and aspirin. *Sixth International Congress of Pharmacology*, Helsinki, July 20–25

Steelman, S. L., Breault, G. O. and Tocco, D. J. (1975). Pharmacokinetics of MK-647 a novel salicylate. *Clin. Pharmacol. Ther.* **17**, 245.

Klotz, J. J. (1966). The Wilcoxon ties and the computer. *J. Am. Stat. Assoc.* **61**, 772

Summary

A randomized double-blind study in ambulatory patients with osteoarthritis of hip and/or knee was conducted, comparing the efficacy and safety of diflunisal 500 mg daily with glafenine 600 mg daily for 4 weeks, followed by an open treatment period with optional increase of dosage to 750 mg diflunisal and 800 mg glafenine respectively.

Thirty patients participated in the study.

The study has shown that diflunisal is superior to glafenine in reducing signs and symptoms associated with osteoarthritis of hip/and or knee.

Zusammenfassung

Es wurde eine wahllose, doppelt blinde Studie an ambulanten Patienten mit Osteoarthritis der Hüfte und/oder des Knies durchgeführt, in der die Wirksamkeit und

Sicherheit von Diflunisal, 500 mg täglich, mit Glafenine, 600 mg täglich, vier Wochen lang verglichen wurde, mit einem anschließenden offenen Behandlungszeitraum mit freigestellter Erhöhung der Dosierung auf 750 mg Diflunisal bzw. 800 mg Glafenine.

Dreißig Patienten (15 je Behandlungsgruppe) im Alter zwischen 36 und 69 Jahren nahmen an dieser Studie teil. Nach einer einwöchigen Placebo-Spüldauer wurden die Patienten wahllos zur Behandlung zugeteilt. Die Patienten wurden ganz zu Beginn und wiederum nach 2, 4 und 8 Wochen Prüftherapie gesehen. Bei jeder Beobachtung wurden gewichtstragender Schmerz, Schwierigkeit mit einer funktionellen Tätigkeit und Nachtschmerz von uns abgeschätzt. Die Dauer der durch Untätigkeit bedingten Steifigkeit in Minuten wurde ebenfalls aufgezeichnet. Außerdem wurde sowohl der Patienten- wie auch der Globaleffekt der Therapie abgeschätzt.

Laboratoriumsbestimmungen wurden in den Wochen 1 und 8 durchgeführt. Abgesehen von einem Patienten in der Diflunisal-Gruppe wurden keine widrigen Reaktionen festgestellt. Die Ergebnisse der Studie haben gezeigt, daß Diflunisal in der Reduzierung der Anzeichen und Symptome in Verbindung mit Osteoarthritis der Hüfte und/oder des Knies dem Glafenine überlegen ist.

Résumé

Une étude aléatorisée à double anonymat est faite sur des malades ambulatoires souffrant d'ostéoarthrite de la hanche et/ou du genou pendant quatre semaines pour comparer l'efficacité et l'innocuité du diflunisal (500 mg par jour) et de la glafénine (600 mg par jour), suivie d'une période de traitement "ouverte avec augmentation facultative de la posologie jusqu'à 750 mg de diflunisal ou 800 mg de glafénine.

Trente malades (quinze par groupe) de 36 à 69 ans participent à l'étude. Après une semaine d'échec de placebo, les malades sont répartis au hasard entre les deux groupes. Les malades sont visités avant le début du traitement et après 2, 4 et 8 semaines du traitement d'essai. A chaque observation, on évalue la douleur de portage de poids, la difficulté d'une activité fonctionnelle et la douleur nocturne. On note aussi la durée de la raideur due à l'inactivité en minutes. En outre, on apprécie le malade et l'effet global du traitement.

Les dosages de laboratoire sont faits aux semaines 1 et 8. Sauf pour un malade du groupe "diflunisal", on ne constate aucune réaction défavorable. Les résultats de l'étude montrent que le diflunisal est supérieur à la glafénine pour atténuer les signes et symptômes liés à l'ostéoarthrite de la hanche et/ou du genou.

Sommario

Su pazienti ambulatoriali con osteoartrite dell'anca e/o ginocchio si condusse, per la durata di quattro settimane, uno studio casualizzato "double-blind" allo scopo di raffrontare l'efficacia e la sicurezza del diflunisal (500 mg/giorno) con quella della glafenine (600 mg/giorno) facendolo poi seguire da un periodo di trattamento aperto con aumento opzionale della dose fino a 750 mg per il diflunisal e 800 mg per la glafenine.

A questo studio parteciparono 30 pazienti (15 per gruppo) con età da 36 a 69 anni. Dopo una settimana di somministrazione di placebo (sostanza innocua a scopo suggestivo) si assegnarono i pazienti al trattamento. Si esaminarono i pazienti alla partenza e quindi dopo 2, 4 e 8 settimane di terapia. A ciascuna osservazione valutammo il dolore a sostenere il peso del corpo, le difficoltà funzionali e i dolori notturni. Si prese pure nota della durata in minuti della rigidità per inattività. Oltre a ciò si valutarono sia i pazienti che l'effetto globale della terapia.

Si esequirono analisi da laboratorio alle settimane 1 e 8. Ad eccezione di un paziente nel gruppo diflunisal, non si osservò alcuna reazione avversa. I risultati dello studio hanno mostrato che il diflunisal è superiore alla glafenine nella riduzione dei sintomi relativi alla osteoartrite dell'anca e/o ginocchio.

Resumen

Se realizó un estudio aleatorio de doble ciego en pacientes ambulatorios con artrosis de cadera y/o rodilla para comparar la eficacia y seguridad del diflunisal (500 mg por día) con la de la glafenina (600 mg por día) durante 4 semanas, seguido de un periodo de tratamiento de tiempo indeterminado con la opción de aumentar la dosis de diflunisal hasta 750 mg y hasta 800 mg la de glafenina.

Participaron en el estudio 30 pacientes (15 en cada grupo de tratamiento), cuyas edades iban de 36 a 69 años. Los pacientes se distribuyeron al azar en dos grupos, leugo de un periodo de una semana de "lavado" con placebo. Los pacientes fueron vistos al comienzo y a las 2, 4 y 8 semanas de la terapia de prueba. En cada obser-observación, calculamos el dolor al soportar peso, la dificultad en actividades funcionales y el dolor nocturno. También se registró la duración en minutos de la rigidez por inactividad. Asimismo, se evaluó el estado del paciente y el efecto global de la terapia.

Se realizaron exámenes de laboratorio en la primera y octava semanas. No se observaron reacciones adversas, excepto en un paciente del grupo de diflunisal. Los resultados del estudio han demostrado que el diflunisal es superior a la glafenina en la reducción de señales y síntomas asociados con la artrosis de cadera y/o rodilla.

Sumário

Um estudo duplamente às cegas e ao acaso foi efectuado em doentes ambulatórios com osteo-artrite da anca e/ou joelho, para comparar a eficácia e grau de segurança do diflunisal (500 mg/dia) com a da glafenina (600 mg/dia), durante quatro semanas, seguidas por um período de tratamento em regime aberto com aumento opcional da dose para 750 mg de diflunisal e 800 mg de glafenina.

Trinta doentes (15 em cada grupo), cuja idade variava entre 36 e 69 anos, participaram neste estudo. Após uma semana de "tempo-morto"—em que os doentes receberam um placebo, para eliminarem quaisquer efeitos de terapêutica precedente— os doentes foram distribuídos ao acaso para fins de tratamento. Os doentes foram observados "à partida" e novamente após 2, 4 e 8 semanas do ensaio terapêutico. Em cada observação, a dor causada pelo pêso do corpo, a dificuldade de actividade funcional e a dor nocturna, foram classificadas em categorias por nós. A duração em minutos da rigidez por inactividade foi também registada. Além disso, foi avaliada a eficácia da terapêutica tanto sob o ponto do doente como de modo global.

Determinações laboratoriais foram feitas ao fim da 1^a e da 8ª semanas. Salvo no caso de um doente no grupo diflunisal, não foram observadas quaisquer reacções adversas. Os resultados do estudo mostraram que o diflunisal é superior à glafenina no que respeita à redução de sinais e sintomas associados com osteo-artrite da anca e/ou joelho.

Double Blind Study of Diflunisal compared with Aspirin in Arthrosis of the Hip and/or Knee: Comparison of Analgesia

J. HONORATO, R. MARTI MASSO and J. AZANZA

*Department of Clinical Pharmacology,
University of Navarre Medical School Clinic, Spain*

J. R. VALENTI AND J. BEQUIRISTAIN

*Orthopedic Surgery and Traumatology Department
University of Navarre Medical School Clinic, Spain*

Diflunisal (5-(4-difluorophenyl) salicylic acid) is a new analgesic and anti-inflammatory agent discovered during screening more than 500 similar compounds. It has been found to have greater potency, better tolerance and a longer lasting effect than other salicylates.

In experimental animals the analgesic activity of diflunisal is between 7·5 and 13 times that of aspirin; in humans it has about twice the activity of aspirin but the effect lasts longer. Considerable anti-inflammatory activity has been shown in carrageenin-induced swelling of the paw in rats and in arthritis. This activity is related to the 5-(4-fluorophenyl) group and is similar to that of pyrazolidines, steroids and phenyl-alkalones. It possesses 1·4 times the anti-pyretic activity of aspirin and is about three times as active in reducing inflammation induced by injecting urate crystals into the knee of the dog.

Diflunisal, when added in high concentrations to *in vitro* platelet test solution will partially inhibit platelet aggregation. However, in clinical tests involving dose regimens as high as 500 mg b.i.d., diflunisal did not have any adverse effects on platelet function tests. Diflunisal on a mg basis, appears to be less potent than aspirin as an inhibitor of prostaglandin synthetase. Clinical testing, however, reveals that therapeutic dose regimens of diflunisal are associated with decreases in urinary prostaglandin E and E_1 metabolite of the same magnitude as the decrease associated with a therapeutic regimen of aspirin or sulindac. The peak serum level of diflunisal is reached 2 h after oral administration, the half-life is about 8 h and some 95% is excreted in the urine with 85–90% as one of two glucuronides. No interaction with other drugs, including oral anti-diabetics, diuretics, analgesics and nonsteroidal anti-inflammatory agents, has been discovered.

Diflunisal: Royal Society of Medicine International Congress and Symposium Series No. 6, published jointly by Academic Press Inc. (London) Ltd., and the Royal Society of Medicine.

Patients and Methods

Twenty subjects (9 men; 11 women) whose ages ranged from 37 to 68 years (average 54·05 years±1·77) were selected in accordance with pre-determined criteria. Eleven were affected mainly in the knee and nine mainly in the hip, although all had symptoms in other joints.

The period for which the subjects had suffered from the disorder ranged from two years to 17 years, the average being 7·95 years±1·03, and there was a consistent picture of severe pain, with varying effects on function. Drugs taken prior to the trial were found to be mainly alkaline derivatives for seven subjects, indole drugs for six, aspirin for three and phenylbutazone for one. The remaining four patients had no recent history of analgesic and/or anti-inflammatory drug treatment.

All patients took part in a double-blind study for 12 weeks being assigned by a pre-determined random selection procedure, to one of two groups; one group receiving aspirin and the other diflunisal. The first 4 weeks were used for dosage adjustment and the subjects took varying doses. Group 1 (diflunisal) started with 250 mg in the morning and 250 mg in the afternoon, with placebo midday and at night; Group II (aspirin) initially received 200 mg in four doses. According to the results in the initial period, the daily dosage was raised, in some cases to up to 750 mg of diflunisal or up to 3 g aspirin.

In weeks 5 to 12 the subjects received the optimum dosage found in the adjustment period, with the result that the mean for diflunisal was 625·0±41·7 mg with five patients receiving 500 mg at the end of the adjustment period and another five taking 750 mg. In the aspirin group eight patients were receiving 2 g at the end of the adjustment period and two patients were on 3 g (mean 2·2±0·33 g).

These dosages were continued from week 12 to week 48 in an open continuation of the trial. The clinical evaluation which was carried out during the trial covered case history, physical examination, biochemical analyses, ECG, tests of hearing and eyesight, X-ray and side-effects. The check-ups were made at the end of the baseline week and in weeks 2, 4, 8 and 12 of the double-blind study and in weeks 16, 20, 24, 32, 40 and 48 of the open period.

The statistical analysis and evaluation of results have been confined to weeks 4, 8, 12, 24 and 48 in order to simplify the report. (We carried out a linear study, using the Wilcoxon rank sum test and a comparative study of the two therapeutic groups by means of the Kruskal–Wallis test.)

Results

Three assessments of pain were used, (1) the subjects' subjective evaluation of the pain, (2) night pain and (3) pain in connection with a specific function which was different for each patient (e.g. tying shoelaces, going up or down stairs or getting into a car).

Evaluation of the Pain

The subject's subjective evaluation of the pain

This was measured in all the subjects from a scale of values from absence of pain (0) to the maximum possible pain (4). The only features of the means in the course of the trial which deserve special mention are the initially higher value of the mean for the diflunisal group in week 0 and the gradual, almost synchronous lowering of the mean for both groups (Fig. 1). Statistical analysis gives levels of significance from weeks 4 to 48 of $P<0.01$ for the diflunisal group and of $P<0.05$ for the aspirin group.

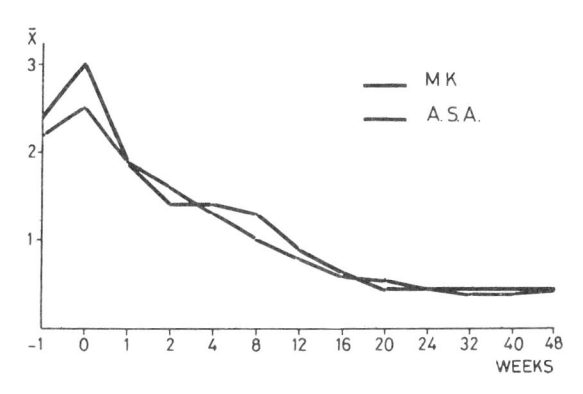

Figure 1. Weight bearing pain—mean evaluation.

Night pain

Each patient was asked at each appointment about the intensity of night pain, which was again evaluated on a scale from 0 to 4 (Fig. 2). All the subjects said at the begin-

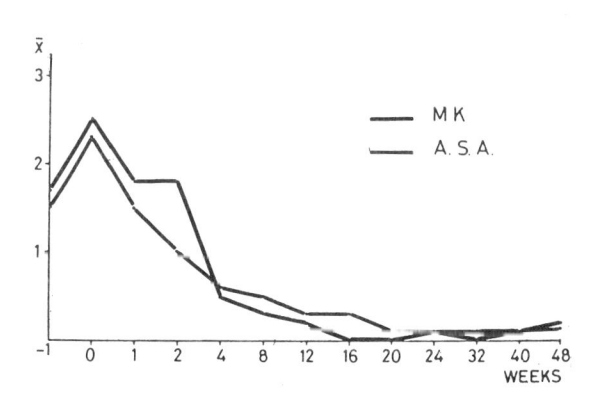

Figure 2. Night pain—mean evaluation.

ning of the trial that they had night pain. The mean values for the two groups at the end of the baseline period were very similar and the lowering almost matched, except in the case of weeks 16, 20 and 32, when none of the subjects in the diflunisal group had night pain. Statistical analysis of the lowering of the means shows very significant change from the sixth week onwards for both groups with $P<0.01$ at the end of the trial.

Difficulty in connection with a specific function

Initially high mean values for both groups were obtained and the figures were slightly higher for the diflunisal group (Fig. 3). The drop was fairly similar and in the diflunisal

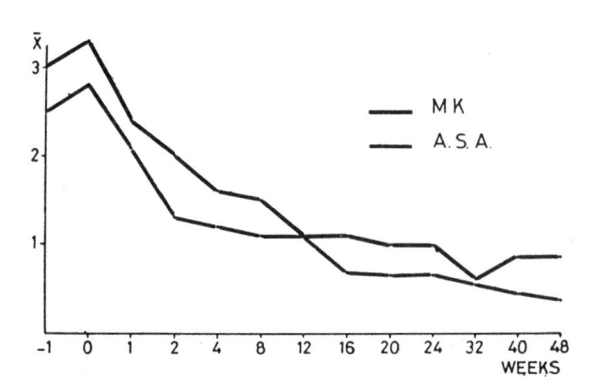

Figure 3. Difficulty in specific function—mean evaluation.

group was significant in the first few weeks ($P<0.05$). From week 4 onwards this level of significance was reached in both groups. In each subject the most painful function was evaluated and was retained for that individual throughout the trial, using a scale of values from 0, for no difficulty, to 4 denoting that the subject needed assistance.

Evaluation from Clinical Features Relating to Inflammation

This set of measurements comprised (1) degree of morning stiffness (2) abduction of the hip for subjects suffering from arthrosis of the hip and (3) flexion of the knee for those affected by arthrosis of the knee.

As this was a trial of an analgesic the subjects were selected because of pain and although it is difficult to separate inflammation and pain in patients of this kind, it can happen, as was the case in the trial, that the parameters relating to inflammation initially give means which are of little validity with large deviations from the standard error or very low means.

Morning stiffness

This was measured in minutes on the days of appointments by the subject and the changes in means and analysis of statistical significance are given in Table 1. The

Table 1

Inactivity stiffness—mean scores

Treatment group	Week					
	0	4	8	12	24	48
Diflunisal	21·5	17·0	11·1^a	11·6^a	2·6^b	5·6^a
N	(10)	(10)	(10)	(10)	(9)	(8)
ASA	58·0	28·0^a	15·2^b	11·5^a	4·2^a	6·9
	(10)	(10)	(10)	(10)	(9)	(8)

Within the indicated group the decrease was significant.
$^a P<0.05$; $^b P<0.01$.

initial gap between the means, with a value of 21·5 for the diflunisal group and of 58·0 for the aspirin group is due to the inclusion of a subject with very severe pain and in whom there was rapid improvement. Hence in the latter group, significance appears in week 4, whereas in the diflunisal group it appears in week 8.

Abduction of the hip

The measurement was made in centimetres in a test in which the hip was moved until pain began to be felt and was performed only in the 11 patients with arthrosis of the hip. It is noteworthy that in the baseline period the means for the two groups are very similar, indicating reasonable reliability for purposes of evaluation. There was a steady rise in the mean for both groups in the course of the trial, although statistically significant difference was obtained in the diflunisal group only, from the fourth week ($P<0.05$).

Flexion of the knee

This was measured by goniometer and recorded in degrees, in subjects with arthrosis of the knee. The improvements in the means were constant but in the group of subjects treated with aspirin the improvement appeared rather earlier and was more consistent, with a value of $P<0.05$ throughout the trial.

Evaluation of Response to Therapy

The patient made a general evaluation of a set of subjective data, including pain, ability to perform movements, ability to walk, etc. The investigator evaluated a set of objective data—morning stiffness, flexion and abduction. The two evaluations are usually very similar in result and the same scale is used: 0 for no improvement at all up to 4 for an excellent response.

Patient's evaluation

Starting from week 4 in the diflunisal group, the response was reported as excellent (one patient), good (five), moderate (two) and poor (two). In the aspirin group the figures were excellent (two), good (three) and moderate (five). Overall there was no marked difference between the two groups except in week 16 when eight subjects (88%) in the diflunisal group came into the area of excellent or good response, compared with 70% in the aspirin group. At the end of the trial both groups had 100% in the area of excellent or good response.

Investigator's evaluation

Using the same scale of values the investigator assessed the quality of the response to therapy and the two evaluations, by the investigator and by the patient, were similar. Thus, the data obtained show that for both therapeutic groups, a 100% of good or excellent response was obtained at the end of 48 weeks.

Side Effects

In assessing the incidence of side-effects it should be remembered that this trial lasted 48 weeks and heavy dosages of both acetylsalicylic acid (ASA) and of diflunisal were used.

In the diflunisal group there was one case of acute gastric ulcer, sited in the greater curvature, with pain for about 2 weeks and leading to copious gastric haemorrhage necessitating partial gastrectomy. Apart from that case, mild epigastric pain developed in another subject on two occasions, the total duration being 22 days. Severe pain, vomiting and nausea were confined to the patient with acute gastric ulcer.

In the aspirin group, two subjects suffered digestive upset, one in the form of mild pain for 2 days and the other with dyspepsia, also mild, lasting 5 days. Another patient showed a typical ASA reaction with pain of moderate intensity, which ceased spontaneously after 18 days. Another patient experienced a mild skin rash for 8 days during the treatment.

Only four subjects dropped out of the trial, two from each group. For two patients, one in each group, the reason was inability to follow-up, another was the patient in the diflunisal group who developed acute ulcer and the fourth was a patient who failed to respond to treatment with aspirin.

No persistent change which could have been caused by either of the drugs was observed at any time during the trial in any of the laboratory tests or examinations carried out.

Discussion

The present trend towards using ASA and its derivatives more and more frequently in clinical practice has arisen not from a return to the medicine of the past but because of various long-term experimental and clinical findings.

Better understanding of the mechanisms giving rise to inflammation, the connection through bioactive polypeptides with the mechanisms of platelet aggregation and fibrin formation, have produced fuller information concerning the mode of action of ASA and its derivatives. Twenty years ago the therapeutic indications were limited to analgesia, anti-pyrexia and combating inflammation but now they have been expanded to take in all disorders in which it is important to inhibit platelet aggregation and prostaglandin synthesis. However, the authors believe that despite the detailed knowledge now available, these preparations still have unsuspected properties.

Another recent finding which permits more rational use of salicylates is the greater specificity of use of each of them, according to the mode of action. Some of the trifluorides are known to be more active against platelet aggregation than as analgesics and anti-inflammatory agents. Other recently discovered preparations display greater potency *in vitro* and *in vivo* than aspirin itself does, not only because of their pharmacological actions but also because of different pharmacodynamic behaviour. Differences in absorption, in the length of time for which they remain in the blood, in metabolism and in elimination make them more useful from the clinical point of view.

Finally, there is a third aspect which is very prominent in all basic research programmes. This is the search for new preparations with the same pharmacokinetic properties but with a lower incidence of iatrogenic effects which occur so frequently with the salicylates. Diflunisal is one compound to emerge from those research programmes.

As a result of the comparative study reported above, lasting for 48 weeks, in patients suffering from osteoarthritis of the hip and/or knee, it can be concluded that diflunisal showed slightly better action than aspirin against subjective pain, night pain and pain in performing a specific function.

As regards the actual effect against inflammation, the results looked more like chance findings than therapeutic evidence. However, both the drugs were active and their activity was reflected in change in the means, except that statistically significant difference was not obtained in the aspirin group for abduction of the hip.

Although there was a strikingly small difference between the two compounds in terms of evaluation of the therapeutic response, responses were obtained with both. Comparative statistical study of the two groups by means of the Kruskal–Wallis tests gave the result of no significant difference in any of the parameters.

Two important aspects emerge from the trial, the small number of drop-outs and the good patient compliance. In connection with the former, it should be remembered that in this country doses of 2–3 g of aspirin frequently cause digestive upset, correlating with the high alcohol intake. As to the latter, it is very difficult to get patients, who feel better, to persist with medication. These aspects enhance the value of our statistical study, because results can be obscured when subjects drop out of a trial as it is always possible that they have not responded to the treatment.

These findings are of some value since they form part of a larger, multi-centre trial and further data will be available in due course to substantiate or refute these preliminary results.

Conclusion

A trial was carried out in 20 subjects (9 men; 11 women) suffering from arthrosis of the hip and/or knee. They were randomly assigned to one of two groups, one of which was treated with diflunisal and the other with aspirin.

In compliance with the pre-arranged methodology for a multicentre trial, periodic check-up was performed until the end of the trial, i.e. after 48 weeks. At each appointment there was subjective evaluation of pain and evaluation of night pain and pain in performing a specific function, also evaluation by objective parameters of stiffness in the morning, abduction of the hip and/or flexion of the knee.

Linear and comparative statistical analysis of the two groups for each of the parameters were produced. The side-effects observed are also reported.

Finally, the usefulness of new preparations of the kind tested is discussed and the conclusions are stated.

Summary

Twenty patients (9 male: 11 female) with osteoarthritis were randomly allocated to one of two groups—diflunisal was given in doses of 250–500 mg and ASA in doses of 2–3 g. After the 4-week titration period, constant dosage was maintained throughout the study.

Assessment of pain was done by Students' t test comparing week 0 with each visit. A significant reduction of weight-bearing pain was noticed in the diflunisal group from week 16, with $P<0.02$ and from week 20 to 48 with $P<0.01$, clearly more distinct than in the group of patients on ASA, where reductions from mean baseline are not statistically significant. Also in night pain where we have significant values ($P<0.02$) on week 4 in the diflunisal group, whereas $P<0.05$ on week 12 with patients on ASA.

Morning stiffness, flexion of knee and abduction were assessed in the same way. The patients' and investigators' opinion on therapeutic effect were assessed in absolute values.

The comparative evaluation of diflunisal and ASA showed a superior therapeutic response in subjective and objective parameters of pain and inflammation, with less side-effects with diflunisal including gastrointestinal signs and symptoms. Electrocardiographic, audiometric and ophthalmological examinations revealed no adverse effects.

We believe that diflunisal, a new longer-acting analgesic, has greater therapeutic activity and lower incidence of side effects than ASA, making it a useful drug in the treatment of inflammatory processes.

Zusammenfassung

Zwanzig Patienten (9 Männer, 11 Frauen) mit Osteoarthritis wurden wahllos einer von zwei Gruppen zugewiesen—Diflunisal wurde in Dosen von 250–500 mg und Azetylsalizylsäure (ASA) in Dosen von 2–3 Gramm verabreicht. Nach der vierwöchigen Titrationszeit wurde während der gesamten Studie eine gleichbleibende Dosierung beibehalten.

Die Abschätzung des Schmerzes erfolgte durch eine Studentenprüfung, in der die Woche O bei jedem Besuch verglichen wurde. In der Diflunisal-Gruppe wurde ab Woche 16 eine Verminderung des gewichtstragenden Schmerzes mit $P<0,02$, und von Woche 20 bis 48 mit $P<0,01$ verzeichnet; das ist eindeutig ausgeprägter als in der Gruppe der Patienten auf ASA, wo Verminderungen von der mittleren Basis statistisch nicht bedeutsam sind. Ebenso im Nachtschmerz, wo wir bedeutsame Werte

($P<0{,}02$) auf Woche 4 in der Gruppe diflunisal haben, hingegen $P<0{,}05$ auf Woche 12 mit Patienten auf ASA.

Morgensteife, Beugung des Knies und Abduktion wurden in derselben Weise abgeschätzt. Die Meinung der Patienten und der Forscher in bezug auf die therapeutische Wirkung wurde in Absolutwerten abgeschätzt.

Die vergleichende Auswertung von Diflunisal und ASA zeigte eine überlegene therapeutische Reaktion in subjektiven und objektiven Parametern von Schmerz und Entzündung, mit weniger Nebenwirkungen bei Diflunisal einschließlich gastrointestinaler Anzeichen und Symptome. Elektrokardiographische, audiometrische und ophthalmologische Untersuchungen ergaben keine nachteiligen Auswirkungen.

Wir glauben, daß Diflunisal—ein neues, länger wirkendes Analgetikum—eine größere therapeutische Wirksamkeit und ein geringeres Auftreten von Nebenwirkungen hat als ASA und dadurch eine nützliche Droge bei der Behandlung von Entzündungsprozessen ist.

Résumé

Vingt malades (9 hommes, 11 femmes) souffrant d'ostéoarthrite sont répartis au hasard en deux groupes, dont l'un reçoit du diflunisal à des doses de 250–500 mg et l'autre de l'acide acétylsalicylique à des doses de 2–3 g. Après la période de dosage de quatre semaines, on maintient les posologies constantes pendant toute l'étude.

La douleur est évaluée par l'essai de Student, en comparant la semaine 0 avec chaque visite. On note une diminution significative de la douleur de portage de poids dans le groupe "diflunisal" à partir de la semaine 16 ($P<0{,}02$) et de la semaine 20 à la semaine 48 ($P<0{,}01$), bien plus nette que dans le groupe "acide acétylsalicylique", où les diminutions à partir de la moyenne initiale ne sont pas statistiquement significatives. Pour la douleur nocturne, on a aussi des valeurs significatives ($P<0{,}02$) la semaine 4 dans le groupe diflunisal, contre $P<0{,}05$ la semaine 12 pour le groupe "acide acétylsalicylique".

La raideur matinale, la flexion du genou et l'adduction ont été vérifiées de la même manière. Les opinions des malades et des chercheurs sur l'effet thérapeutique ont été établies en valeur absolue.

L'évaluation comparative du diflunisal et de l'acide acétylsalicylique montre une meilleure réaction thérapeutique (paramètres subjectifs et objectifs) de la douleur et de l'inflammation, avec des effets secondaires bien moindres pour le diflunisal, y compris les signes et symptômes gastro-intestinaux. Les examens électrocardiographiques, audiométriques et ophtalmologiques ne révèlent pas d'effets nocifs.

Nous pensons que le diflunisal, nouvel analgésique à action prolongée, a un effet thérapeutique plus grand et des effets secondaires moindres que l'acide acétylsalicylique, ce qui en fait un médicament utile dans le traitement des processus inflammatoires.

Sommario

Si ripartirono casualmente venti pazienti affetti da osteoartrite (9 maschi e 11 femmine) in due gruppi somministrando diflunisal in dosi di 250–500 mg ai pazienti di un gruppo e acido acetilsalicilico (AAS) in dosi di 2–3 grammi a quelli dell'altro. Dopo il periodo di titolazione durato quattro settimane, si mantenne una dose costante per il resto dello studio.

L'effetto analgesico venne valutato mettendo a raffronto la settimana 0 con ciascuna visita. Si notò una notevole riduzione dei dolori con giunto sottocarico nel gruppo diflunisal a partire dalla settimana 16 con $P<0,02$ e della settimana 20 alla 48 con $P<0,01$, riduzione chiaramente più distinta che nel gruppo AAS, in cui questa non si scostò dal valore medio di partenza in modo statisticamente significativo. Pure nel caso dei dolori notturni dove abbiamo valori significativi ($P<0,02$) alla settimana 4 del gruppo diflunisal, mentre $P<0,05$ alla settimana 12 con i pazienti del gruppo AAS.

Nel medesimo modo si valutarono la rigidità mattutina, flessione e adduzione del ginocchio. Le opinioni sugli effetti terapeutici da parte dei pazienti e indagatori vennero tradotte in valori assoluti.

Queste prove comparative hanno mostrato che il diflunisal offre una risposta terapeutica superiore nei parametri analgesici e antiflogistici sia soggettivi che obiettivi, con minori effetti secondari compresi quelli gastro-intestinali. Gli esami elettrocardiografici, audiometrici e oftalmologici non rivelarono alcun effetto avverso.

Siamo dell'opinione che il diflunisal, un nuovo analgesico con azione prolungata, abbia un maggior effetto terapeutico e una minor incidenza di effetti secondari dell'AAS, ciò che lo rende quindi un farmaco molto utile nel trattamento di affezioni infiammatorie.

Resumen

Se distribuyeron 20 pacientes (9 de sexo masculino y 11 de sexo femenino) al azar en dos grupos con artrosis—el diflunisal se dio en dosis de 250–500 mg y el ácido acetilsalicílico (AAS) en dosis de 2 a 3 g. Luego de un perido de dosificación de 4 semanas, se mantuvieron dosis constantes durante todo el estudio.

El dolor se evaluó con el test de estudiantes, comparando la semana O con cada visita. Se observó una reducción considerable en el dolor provocado por el peso, con el grupo de diflunisal, a partir de la decimosexta semana con $P<0,02$ y, de las semanas 20 a 48, con $P<0,01$, resultados éstos evidentemente más acentuados que los del grupo de pacientes con AAS, cuyas reducciones a partir de los valores iniciales no tienen importancia estadística. Asimismo, para el dolor nocturno se obtuvieron valores importantes ($P<0,02$) en el grupo del diflunisal a la cuarta semana y sólo valores de $P<0,05$ en los pacientes sometidos a AAS en la duodécima semana.

Se evaluaron de la misma manera la rigidez matinal, la flexión de rodilla y la abducción. La opinión de los pacientes e investigadores acerca del efecto terapéutico se estimó en valores absolutos.

La evaluación comparativa del diflunisal y el AAS demostró que el diflunisal posee una respuesta terapéutica superior para los parámetros subjetivos y objetivos de dolor e inflamación y menor incidencia de efectos secundarios, incluyendo síntomas y señales gastrointestinales. Los exámenes electrocardiográficos, audiométricos y oftalmológicos no revelaron ningún efecto perjudicial.

Estamos convencidos que el diflunisal, como nuevo analgésico de acción prolongada, posee mayor actividad terapéutica y menor incidencia de efectos secundarios que el AAS, lo cual hace que se considere como un medicamento útil para el tratamiento de procesos inflamatorios.

Sumário

Vinte doentes (9 homens e 11 mulheres) com osteo-artrite foram distribuídos, ao acaso, a um de dois grupos de tratamento—diflunisal em doses de 250–500 mg e ácido acetilsalicílico (ASA) em doses de 2–3 g. A partir da quarta semana do período de titulação, foi mantida uma dose constante durante todo o estudo.

A avaliação da dor foi feita pelo teste t de Students, comparando a semana O com cada visita. Uma redução significativa da dor causada pelo pêso do corpo foi notada no grupo diflunisal a partir da 16ª semana (com $P<0,02$) e da 20ª até à 48ª semana (com $P<0,01$), sensìvelmente mais distinta do que no grupo ASA onde as reduções de dor a partir da linha média inicial não tiveram significado estatístico. Também em dores nocturnas, registaram-se valores significativos ($P<0,02$) na 4ª semana no grupo diflunisal, ao passo que nos doentes do grupo ASA o valor foi de $P<0,05$ na semana 12.

A rigidez matutina, flexão do joelho e abdução foram avaliadas da mesma maneira. A opinião dos doentes e dos investigadores quanto ao efeito terapêutico foi avaliada em valores absolutos.

A avaliação comparativa do diflunisal e do ASA mostrou uma resposta terapêutica superior em parâmetros subjectivos e objectivos de dor e inflamação, com menos efeitos secundários no caso do diflunisal incluindo perturbações e sintomas gastro-intestinais. Os exames electrocardiográfico, audiométrico e oftalmológico não revelaram quaisquer efeitos secundários.

Cremos, pois, que o diflunisal—um novo analgésico de acção prolongada—tem maior actividade terapêutica e menor incidência de efeitos secundários do que o ASA, o que o torna uma útil droga para o tratamento de processos inflamatórios.

Diflunisal in Minor Surgery

H. L. F. BROM

*Surgical Department, University Hospital,
Leiden, The Netherlands**

Diflunisal is a non-addictive, salicylic acid derived analgesic which has been shown in several studies to have a high degree of efficacy in the relief of pain, with a long duration of action and good tolerance. In addition, diflunisal does not interfere with blood clotting and, as this is a highly desirable property in any analgesic to be used post-operatively, a study was initiated in patients undergoing minor surgical procedures at the University Hospital in Leiden.

Patients and Methods

Patients complaining of pain 60 min or more post-operation were admitted to the study. The surgical procedures included contusions, luxations and fractures, re-setting fractures and various other minor but painful operations. If necessary local anaesthesia was induced using 5–10 ml of 0·5–2% lidocaine.

The trial was an open-controlled randomized investigation to compare the efficacy and tolerance of diflunisal versus glafenine. On entry patients were randomly assigned allocation numbers and following surgery they received an envelope bearing that number, which contained a numbered card corresponding to their assigned allocation number. Attached to the patient cards in the diflunisal group were three envelopes each containing two diflunisal 250 mg tablets. Attached to patient cards in the glafenine group were six envelopes, envelope No. 1 contained two glafenine 200 mg tablets and evelopes 2–6 contained one tablet of 200 mg each.

Patients were instructed to take the first dose of medication at least 1 h after the surgical procedure or later and if no pain developed these patients were excluded from the trial. This was done in order to diminish the influence of the local anaesthesia upon the perception of pain. The subsequent doses were to be taken as needed for pain but patients on diflunisal had to wait 6 h between doses while patients on glafenine had to wait 4 h between doses. Patients were further instructed to record the time each dose was taken as well as the intensity of spontaneous pain on their cards

*Head. Professor Dr. M. Vink.

(none, mild, moderate, severe or very severe). The patients were instructed to take the medication following the guide lines and had to return with their remaining cards for a final evaluation one or two days following the surgical procedure. At this visit the intensity of spontaneous pain as well as the patients' opinion on treatment efficacy was recorded according to the scale mentioned before. The adverse reactions, if present, were then recorded. The investigator's evaluation was noted taking into account the expected spontaneous course of symptoms for the individual patient.

Results

The two groups formed by 80 patients (age 18–64 years) did not differ statistically significantly with regards to any characteristics such as sex, age, etc. The number of dosages of test medication taken by the patients in each treatment group showed that in the diflunisal group 14 (35%) of the patients took only the first dose, while in the glafenine group three patients (8%) only took the first dose. This difference was statistically significant ($P<0.05$). Two patients dropped out of the diflunisal group; one being mentally labile with an extremely low pain threshold. The other did not take the second dose of test medication because he did not believe in the drug. Patients who took only the first dose of test medication had their final evaluation at least 10 h after the intake of the last tablet. This indicates that premature evaluation was not made since 10 h had elapsed after the intake of the last tablet. In both treatment groups the time between surgery and the first dose was similar. However, the time between surgery and the last dose was significantly longer in the glafenine group than in the diflunisal group ($P<0.01$) and the time between surgery and the final evaluation was also significantly longer in the glafenine group, ($P<0.01$).

In the patient's evaluation of the treatment efficacy, there was no statistically significant difference between the treatment groups. However, the total number of patients who recorded excellent and good results favours diflunisal in comparison with glafenine (Fig. 1). The same positive effect for diflunisal can also be seen in the investigator's evaluation of treatment efficacy (Fig. 2). No statistically significant differences between the treatment groups were noted in the evaluation of the adverse side-effects.

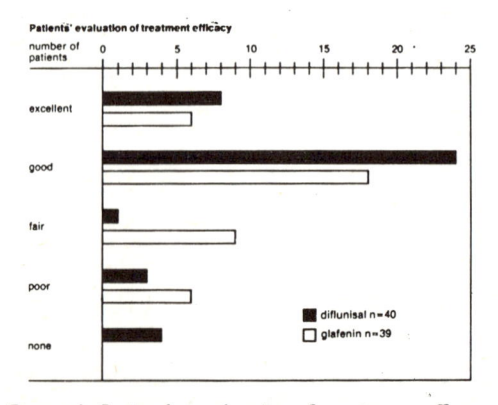

Figure 1. Patient's evaluation of treatment efficacy.

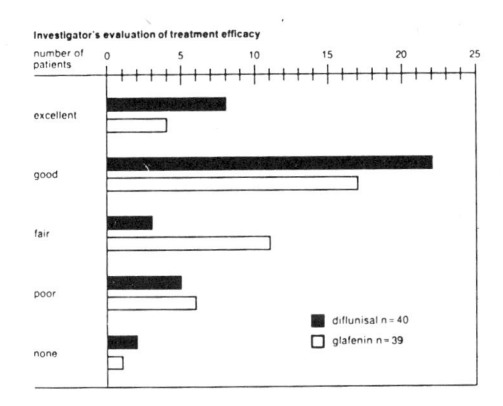

Figure 2. Investigator's evaluation of treatment efficacy.

Conclusions

From the study it is evident that diflunisal relieved pain as well as, or better than, glafenine. The treatment period with diflunisal was shorter than with glafenine with fewer tablets. Because of its long duration of action, diflunisal overcomes breakthrough pain at night and it may be useful in the treatment of fractures.

Summary

An open-controlled randomized study was conducted with diflunisal versus glafenine comparing the efficacy and tolerance of both drugs, in the short-term (1·5 days) relief of pain following minor surgical procedures. Only patients complaining of pain following surgery were included in this study. Eighty patients participated (41 in the diflunisal group and 39 in the glafenine group) with ages ranging from 18–64 years. The initial dose of diflunisal was 500 mg, followed by two additional doses of 500 mg each, administered p.r.n. pain. The initial dose of glafenine was 400 mg, followed by five additional doses of 200 mg p.r.n. pain. The intensity of spontaneous pain was recorded at the final evaluation as well as the patients' opinion on treatment efficacy. The investigator's overall evaluation of efficacy and tolerance of the respective analgesics was recorded.

The results of the study have revealed no statistically significant differences in the degree of pain relief between the treatment groups at the final evaluation. However, the number of patients who required only one dose for pain relief was significantly greater ($P > 0.05$) in the diflunisal group compared to the glafenine group. The persistence of pain following diflunisal treatment was of shorter duration compared to glafenine treatment. No significant adverse reactions were observed in either of the treatment groups.

Zusammenfassung

Es wurde eine offene, kontrollierte, wahllose Studie "Diflunisal gegen Glafenine" durchgeführt, in der die Wirksamkeit und Verträglichkeit beider Drogen in der kurzfristigen (1,5 Tage) Linderung von Schmerz nach kleineren chirurgischen Eingriffen verglichen wurde. In diese Studie wurden nur solche Patienten eingeschlossen, die über Schmerz nach einem chirurgischen Eingriff klagten. Es beteiligten sich achtzig Patienten (41 in der Diflunisal-Gruppe, und 39 in der Glafenine-Gruppe) im Alter zwischen 18 und 64 Jahren. Die Anfangsdosis Diflunisal betrug 500 mg, gefolgt von zwei zusätzlichen Dosen von je 500 mg, die je nach Heftigkeit des Schmerzes verabreicht wurden. Die Anfangsdosis Glafenine betrug 400 mg, gefolgt von 5 zusätzlichen Dosen von 200 mg je nach Heftigkeit des Schmerzes. Die Intensität des Spontanschmerzes wurde bei der Endauswertung ebenso aufgezeichnet wie die Meinung der Patienten über die Wirksamkeit der Behandlung. Die Gesamtauswertung der Wirksamkeit und Verträglichkeit durch den Forscher hinsichtlich der jeweiligen schmerzlindernden Mittel wurde aufgezeichnet.

Die Ergebnisse der Studie haben keine statistisch bedeutsamen Unterschiede in dem Ausmaß der Schmerzlinderung zwischen den Behandlungsgruppen bei der Endauswertung offenbart. Die Zahl der Patienten, die jeweils nur eine Dosis zur Schmerzlinderung benötigten, war jedoch in der Diflunisal-Gruppe bedeutend größer ($P>0.05$) als in der Glafenine-Gruppe. Die Fortdauer des Schmerzes im Anschluß an die Diflunisal-Behandlung war im Vergleich zur Glafenine-Behandlung kürzer. In keiner der beiden Behandlungsgruppen wurden bedeutsame, widrige Reaktionen festgestellt.

Résumé

On fait une étude aléatorisée "ouverte" contrôlée sur le diflunisal et la glafénine pour comparer l'efficacité et la tolérance des deux médicaments dans le soulagement à court terme (1,5 jour) de la douleur après une petite intervention chirurgicale.

Cette étude ne porte que sur des malades se plaignant de douleurs après une opération. 80 malades de 18 à 64 ans participent à l'étude (41 dans le groupe "diflinisal", 39 dans le groupe "glafénine"). La dose initiale de diflunisal est de 500 mg, suivie de deux doses de 500 mg (une à chaque réapparition de la douleur). La dose initiale de glafénine est de 400 mg, suivie de deux doses de 200 mg (une à chaque réapparition de la douleur). On enregistre l'intensité de la douleur spontanée ainsi que l'opinion des malades sur l'efficacité du traitement. On note aussi l'évaluation globale du chercheur sur l'efficacité et la tolérance des deux analgésiques.

Les résultats de l'étude ne révèlent aucune différence statistiquement significative entre les degrés de soulagement de la douleur pour les deux groupes de traitement. Toutefois, le nombre de malades qui n'exigent qu'une seule dose pour être soulagés est significativement plus élevé dans le groupe "diflunisal" que dans le groupe "glafénine". La persistance de la douleur est plus courte après traitement au diflunisal qu'après traitement à la glafénine. On n'observe aucune réaction défavorable significative dans aucun des deux groupes.

Sommario

Si è condotto uno studio casualizzato, controllato e aperto, per raffrontare l'efficacia e tolleranza del diflunisal con la glafenine per analgesia a breve termine (1,5 giorni) dopo piccoli interventi chirurgici. Venero inclusi nello studio soltanto pazienti che presentavano dolori in seguito ad intervento chirurgico. Parteciparono 80 pazienti (41 nel gruppo diflunisal e 39 nel gruppo glafenine) con età dai 18 ai 64 anni. La dose iniziale del diflunisal fu di 500 mg seguita da due ulteriori dosi di 500 mg ciascuna, se dettate dal caso. La dose iniziale della glafenina fu di 400 mg seguita da 5 ulteriori dosi di 200 mg se dettate dal caso. Alla valutazione finale si prese nota dell'intensità dei dolori spontanei nonchè dell'opinione del paziente circa l'efficacia del trattamento. Si prese nota pure del giudizio generale da parte degli indagatori circa l'efficacia e tolleranza dei due analgesici.

I risultati dello studio non hanno rivelato alcuna differenza statisticamente significativa per quanto riguarda il grado di analgesia tra i due gruppi. Tuttavia il numero di pazienti per i quali fu necessaria una sola dose per alleviare il dolore è stato significativamente maggiore ($P>0,05$), nel gruppo diflunisal che nel gruppo glafenine. La persistenza dei dolori dopo il trattamento con diflunisal fu di durata inferiore rispetto alla glafenine. Non si osservarono alcune reazioni avverse significative in nessuno dei due gruppi.

Resumen

Se realizó un estudio libre controlado al azar con diflunisal y glafenina para comparar la eficacia y tolerancia de ambos medicamentos en el alivio del dolor a corto plazo (un día y medio) después de operaciones quirúrgicas de menor importancia. Sólo se incluyeron en este estudio los pacientes que se quejaron de dolor después de la cirugía. Participaron 80 pacientes (41 en el grupo de diflunisal y 39 en el de glafenina), con edades que variaban desde 18 a 64 años. La dosis inicial de diflunisal fue de 500 mg, seguida de dos dosis adicionales opcionales de 500 mg cada una, administradas cuando el paciente manifestaba dolor. La dosis inicial de glafenina fue de 400 mg, seguida de 5 dosis adicionales opcionales de 200 mg ad libitum. Se registró la intensidad del dolor espontáneo en la evaluación final y, asimismo, la opinión del paciente sobre la eficacia del tratamiento. También se registró la opinión general de los investigadores acerca de la eficacia y tolerancia de los respectivos analgésicos.

Los resultados del estudio no revelaron diferencias de importancia estadística entre los dos grupos respecto al grado de alivio del dolor en la evaluación final. Sin embargo, el número de pacientes que sólo necesitaron una dosis ad libitum para alivio del dolor fue bastante mayor en el grupo del diflunisal en comparación con el de la glafenina. La persistencia del dolor luego del tratamiento con diflunisal fue de menor duración que con glafenina. No se observó ninguna reacción adversa en el tratamiento de cualquiera de los grupos.

Sumário

Um estudo aberto, controlado e distribuído ao acaso, foi efectuado com diflunisal e glafenina, comparando a eficácia e tolerância de ambas as drogas, no alívio a curto-prazo (1,5 dias) de dor após pequenas intervenções cirúrgicas. Neste estudo só foram incluídos doentes que se queixaram de dor após intervenção cirúrgica. Ao todo participaram oitenta doentes (41 no grupo diflunisal e 39 no grupo glafenina), de 18–64 anos de idade. A dose inicial de diflunisal foi de 500 mg, seguida por duas doses adicionais de 500 mg cada uma e administradas conforme a necessidade imposta pela dor. A dose inicial de glafenina foi de 400 mg, seguida por 5 doses adicionais de 200 mg administradas conforme a necessidade imposta pela dor. A intensidade de dor espontânea foi registada à avaliação final, bem como a opinião do doente sobre a eficácia do tratamento. A avaliação global feita pelo investigador quanto à eficácia e tolerância dos respectivos analgésicos também foi registada.

Os resultados do estudo não revelaram quaisquer differenças estatìsticamente significativas no grau de alívio de dor entre os dois grupos de tratamento, na altura da avaliação final. Contudo, o número de doentes que necessitaram apenas de 1 dose para aliviar a dor foi significativamente maior ($P>0,05$) no grupo diflunisal do que no grupo glafenina. A persistência de dor após tratamento com diflunisal foi de menor duração comparado com o tratamento com glafenina. Não se observaram quaisquer reacções adversas em nenhum dos grupos de tratamento.

The Analgesic and Anti-Inflammatory Efficacy of Diflunisal compared with Codeine following Removal of Impacted Third Molars

J. K. PETERSEN

Department of Oral Surgery,
The Royal Dental College,
Aarhus, Denmark

Surgical removal of impacted third molars presents a special challenge as the procedure will quite often result in swelling of the cheek and post-operative pain. Aspirin or aspirin-containing combinations have previously been used to relieve pain, but recent studies (Hepsø *et al.*, 1976; Moroz, 1977) have shown that the anti-coagulant effect of aspirin can result in post-operative bleeding and haematoma. The search for new effective analgesics without unwanted effects on the coagulation mechanism has therefore been intensified. One such recent development is diflunisal (Smit-Sibinga, 1977). The efficacy of diflunisal on pain in oral surgery after removal of impacted third molars has previously been documented (Petersen, 1978). The aim of the present study was to compare the analgesic and anti-inflammatory effects of diflunisal as a peripherally acting agent with that of codeine phosphate, which is a centrally acting analgesic, and with that of lactose as a placebo.

Materials and Methods

A method of recording post operative swelling and muscular function of the muscles of mastication has previously been described (Petersen, 1975). By this method the maximum opening distance between the cutting edges of the left central upper and central lower incisor is measured with a ruler. The cheek swelling expressing post-operative oedema and haematoma is registered by applying a facebow with a ruler and a waxbite index that secures accurate repositioning of the apparatus during ensuing registrations. The study design was randomized and double-blind. To 90 patients, in three test groups of 30 patients, the age and sex distribution of whom is seen in Table 1, diflunisal 500 mg b.i.d., codeine phosphate 25 mg q.i.d., and lactose as placebo were administered according to a "double-dummy" schedule as shown in Table 2. The first dosage was given 30 min prior to surgery. Besides the test medica-

---

Diflunisal: Royal Society of Medicine International Congress and Symposium Series No. 6, published jointly by Academic Press Inc. (London) Ltd., and the Royal Society of Medicine.

Table 1

Age and sex distribution of the 90 patients

	Diflunisal	Codeine	Placebo
Age (years)	26.4	24.1	26.4
Range	(19–59)	(18–42)	(19–48)
Male	19	11	13
Female	11	19	17

Numbers in parentheses under age refer to range.

Table 2

Administration of test medication to the three patient groups (double dummy—method: always 2 tablets)

		30 min pre-op.	4 h later	at 18.00 h	at 22.00 h
Day 0	Diflunisal	2×D	2×D	2×P	2×D
	Codeine	1×C, 1×P	2×C	1×C, 1×P	1×C, 1×P
	Placebo	2×P	2×P	2×P	2×P

		at 8.00 h	at 13.00 h	at 18.00 h	at 22.00 h
Day 1–2	Diflunisal	2×D	2×P	2×P	2×D
	Codeine	1×C, 1×P	1×C, 1×P	1×C, 1×P	1×C, 1×P
	Placebo	2×P	2×P	2×P	2×P

		at 8.00 h	at 13.00 h
Day 3	Diflunisal	2×D	2×P
	Codeine	1×C, 1×P	1×C, 1×P
	Placebo	2×P	2×P

D: 1 tablet of 250 mg diflunisal.
C: 1 tablet of 25 mg codeine phosphate + 300 mg (OH)$_9$.
P: 1 tablet of lactose.

tion, which was handed out in envelopes, the patients were supplied with a "reserve analgesic" consisting of 25 tablets of paracetamol 0.5 g. They were allowed to take this reserve analgesic in the event of continuous and severe pain despite the intake of test medication, which was to be taken as ordered in all cases. The patients were asked to record the time and number of intake of paracetamol tablets.

The type of surgery performed on the 90 patients is shown in Table 3. In 17 cases in the diflunisal group, in 17 cases in the codeine group and in 12 cases in the placebo group, the ipsilateral upper third molar was also removed. It is possible to grade the surgical procedure with regard to surgical trauma. In this connection, the duration of surgery from time of incision to the placement of the last suture is the single most important factor. Other factors of importance are the number and shape of roots, the position of the tooth in the jawbone, and the amount of bone to be removed. On the basis of these factors, it is possible to classify the degree of surgical trauma in groups

Table 3

Distribution of surgical procedures in 90 patients

	Diflunisal	Codeine	Placebo
Lower M_3			
Impacted	14	21	15
Semi-Impacted	16	9	15
Lower M_3+Upper M_3	17	17	12

M_3 refers to the third molar, upper, the maxilla and lower, the mandible. Impacted means completely covered by oral mucosa and/or jawbone. Semi-impacted means that there is a break in the mucosal cover.

Table 4

Distribution of degree of surgical trauma among 90 patients and average duration of surgery (min).

		Diflunisal	Codeine	Placebo
Mild	I	4	3	3
Moderate	II	15	16	12
Severe	III	8	9	11
Very severe	IV	3	2	4
Duration of surgery (min)		12·6	12·7	15·0

Table 5

Parameters registered during the study by the investigator (I) and by the patient (P)

Clinical measurements	Day 0	Day 1	Day 3	Day 7
Severity of spontaneous pain	P	P	P	P
Maximal pain since previous visit	—	P	P	—
Degree of pain relief	P	P	P	—
Pain on chewing	P	P	P	P
Ability to sleep	P	P	P	—
Swelling, degree	—	I	I	I
Swelling, facebow	—	I	I	I
Trismus	—	I	I	I
Degree of haematoma	—	I	I	I
Patient's assessment of efficacy	—	P	P	I
Investigator's assessment of efficacy	—	—	—	I

from mild degree (I) to very severe degree (IV) (Table 4). This classification is, of course, important to eliminate bias, when comparing groups.

The clinical measurements listed in Table 5 were registered or recorded. All the patients were operated on and followed by the same investigator, the post-operative checks being on day 1, day 3, and day 7. The recordings on day 0 were done by the patients at home following surgery. For age, duration of surgery, trismus and swelling by facebow measurements, differences among the three treatment groups were assessed by the Kurskall–Wallis test. Pair-wise comparisons between treatment groups were evaluated by Dunn's procedure. For the remaining parameters, differences among the three treatment groups were assessed by the Chi-square test. Pair-wise comparison between treatment groups were evaluated by a $2 \times N$ test for ordered contingency tables or by Fisher's exact test.

Results

Statistical analyses revealed no differences among the three test groups with regard to age and sex distribution, surgical procedure, degree of surgical trauma, duration of surgery, and amount of local analgesic used. Table 6 lists the number of patients with good or excellent pain relief taking no reserve analgesic. They are registered as patients with adequate pain relief. On day 1, diflunisal has a statistically significant better degree of pain relief than codeine and placebo ($P<0.01$). On day 3 there is no statistical difference among the agents.

Table 6

Distribution of patients with adequate pain relief on day 0, day 1, and day 3 post-operatively

Day	Diflunisal	Codeine	Placebo
0	19/30 (63%)	10/30 (33%)[a]	11/30 (37%)
1	23/30 (77%)	12/30 (40%)[b]	9/30 (30%)[b]
3	23/30 (77%)	17/30 (57%)	14/30 (47%)
overall	18/30 (77%)	9/30 (30%)	9/30 (30%)[a]

[a] $P<0.05$.
[b] $P<0.01$.

Interestingly enough, there is no difference between codeine and placebo in the overall score whereas diflunisal is statistically significantly better than both codeine and placebo at the 5% level. Although the mean post-operative swelling in mm as seen to the right in Fig. 1, is less for diflunisal in comparison with codeine and placebo the difference is not statistically significant on any day. If swelling is expressed graphically as a percentage of patients with none or mild degree of swelling, it is seen that the curves of codeine and placebo are very similar (Fig. 2). In addition the largest difference between diflunisal and the other two groups is on day 1, whereafter the curves converge.

The opening ability decreased less with diflunisal than with codeine and placebo (Fig. 3), the difference being statistically significant at the 5% level on day 1. Again, it is noteworthy that the curves of codeine and placebo are almost identical. The number of patients with moderate, severe and very severe degree of post-operative haematoma is also shown in Fig. 3. Less haematoma is found with diflunisal, al-

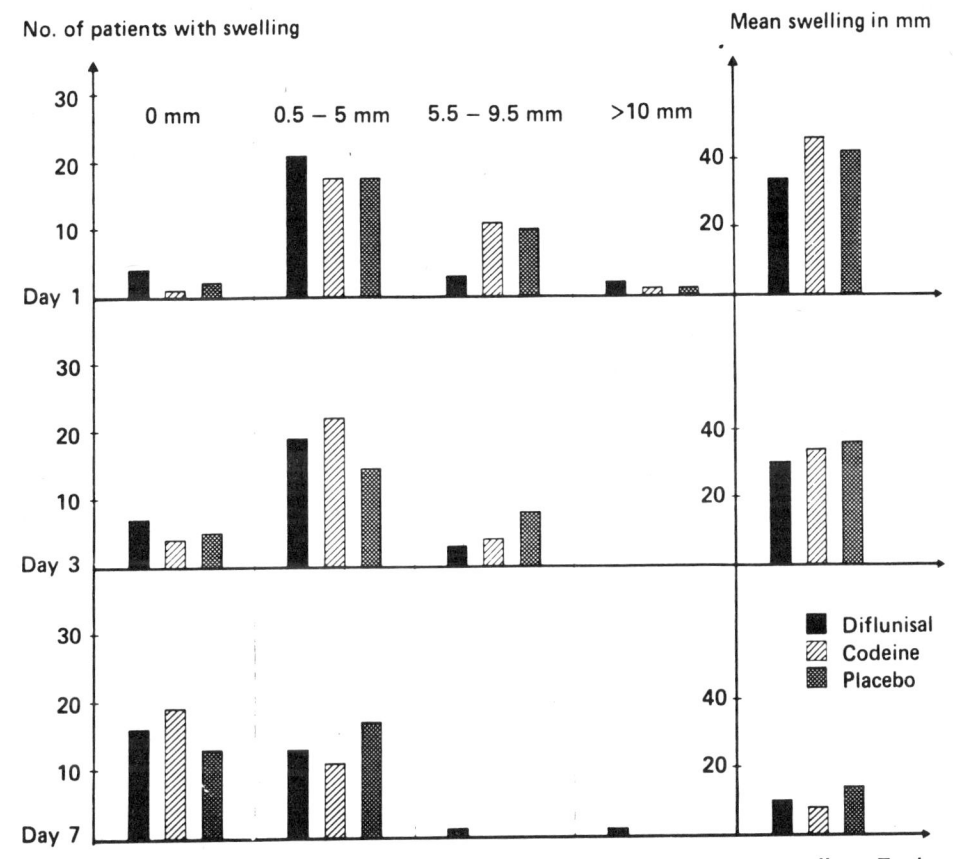

Figure 1. The distribution of patients with different degree of post-operative swelling. To the right the average swelling in mm is given for each test group on days 1, 3, and 7.

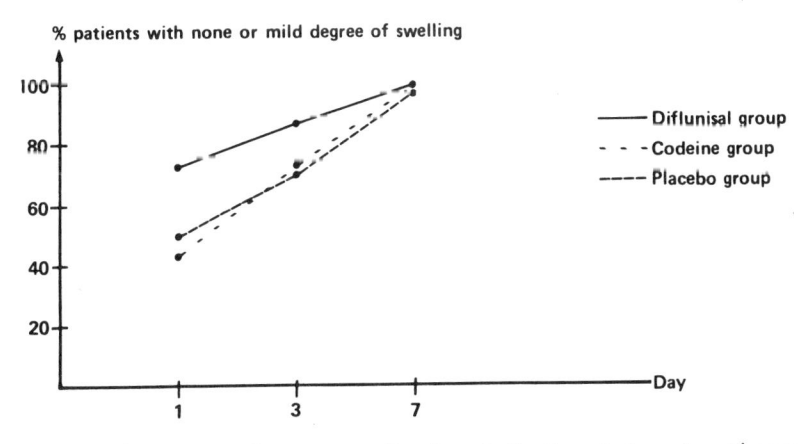

Figure 2. Graphical expression of percentage of patients in the three test groups with none or mild degree of swelling.

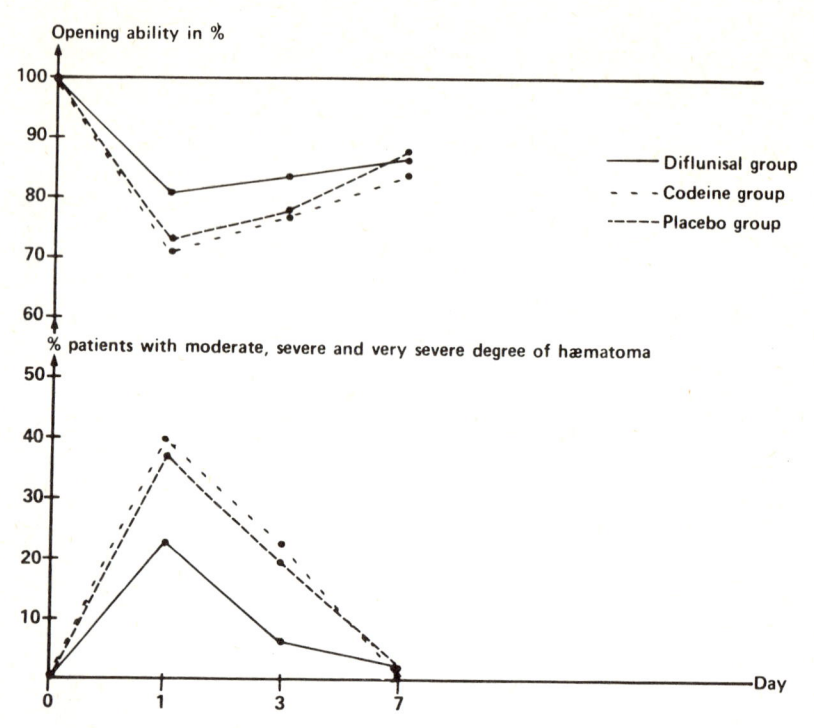

Figure 3. Upper portion: the post-operative maximal opening ability as measured between the incisors in percentage of the pre-operative values. Lower portion: the percentage of patients with moderate, severe and very severe degree of haematoma post-operatively.

though the difference this time is not statistically significant. Again, codeine and placebo seem to parallel, and as has been shown several times, the maximum effect is always on the first post-operative day.

The patients were asked about their ability to sleep as it was thought that severe pain could interfere with normal sleep (Table 7). Only one patient in the diflunisal

Table 7

The ability to sleep post-operatively

Evening of	Sleep disturbed by pain	Diflunisal	Codeine	Placebo
Day 0	yes	0	6 (5)	6 (4)
	no	30 (6)	24 (5)	24 (7)
Day 1	yes	0	5 (4)	7 (5)
	no	30 (5)	25 (1)	23 (3)
Day 2	yes	1 (1)	2 (2)	6 (5)
	no	29 (3)	28 (3)	24 (2)

Numbers in parentheses refer to patients taking the reserve analgesic besides test medication.

Table 8
The type and incidence of adverse reactions listed as numbers of patients

	Diflunisal	No. of patients Codeine	Placebo
CNS			
Headache		1	2
Dizziness		2	
Sleepiness	2	4	1
Insomnia	1		
G-I-tract			
Constipation		2	
Nausea		2	2
Dyspepsia		1	
Diarrhoea			1
Others			
Pruritus		1	
Fatigue	3	2	3
Total	6 = 20%	12 = 40%	8 = 27%

group had sleep disturbance on day 2. Diflunisal had a statistically significantly better sleep score on the evening of day 0 and day 1 than codeine and placebo ($P<0.05$).

The incidence and type of adverse reactions are listed in Table 8. The incidence was less for diflunisal compared with that of codeine and placebo, but the difference was not statistically significant. The total score at the bottom line is less than the added cases, as several patients had more than one adverse reaction. In no case were the adverse reactions serious nor did they lead to the patient's discontinuance of drug intake. The criteria for adequacy of treatment are the patient's evaluation of excellent or good effect with no additional analgesic taken. Inadequate treatment involves a pain efficacy rating of fair, poor or none, and/or intake of reserve analgesic (Table 9). The difference noted on day 1 is statistically significantly in favour of diflunisal at the 5% level. On day 3 the observed difference is no longer significant.

If the incidence of adverse reactions is added to the criteria of adequate treatment mentioned previously, the results are as shown on the bar diagram in Fig. 4. Success is defined as patient evaluation of excellent or good effect, no additional analgesic

Table 9
The distribution of patients with regard to adequacy of treatment according to patients' assessment

		Diflunisal	Codeine	Placebo
Day 1	Adequate	23	14	13
	Inadequate	7	16	17
Day 3	Adequate	23	19	17
	Inadequate	7	11	13

taken, and no adverse reactions recorded. There was no significant difference among the treatment groups in the proportion of patients with a success of treatment. It is remarkable that placebo had so many cases of success as was actually found (12 patients = 40%).

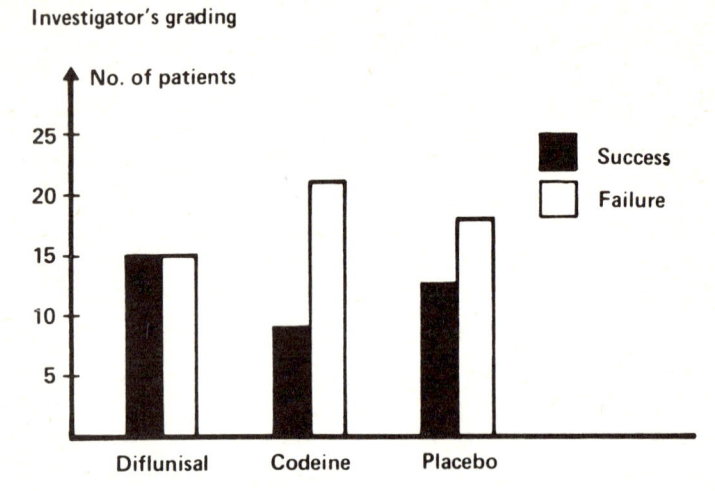

Figure 4. Distribution of number of patients with success or failure of test medication according to investigator's grading and criteria in text.

A presentation of the number of paracetamol tablets taken as reserve analgesic tablets, revealed a large increase in tablet consumption after day 3 in the diflunisal group (Fig. 5). This is caused by severe pain starting on day 2–4 in some patients. This is due to a condition known as "dry socket" or alveolitis sicca dolorosa. Analysis of distribution of dry socket showed that there were 10 patients or 33% in the diflunisal group who developed this complication (Fig. 6). As only two and one in the codeine and placebo groups respectively developed this complication, the difference between diflunisal and the other groups is highly statistically significant ($P<0.01$).

Discussion

The results demonstrate that diflunisal is an effective analgesic in comparison to codeine phosphate and placebo in the treatment of pain following removal of impacted third molars. The analgesic effect of diflunisal is significant on the first post-operative day, but then the superiority over codeine and placebo seems to disappear over the following days. Codeine is a centrally acting analgesic which is demethylated to morphine in the liver and acts via the opiate receptors in the central nervous system. Diflunisal on the other hand is a peripherally acting analgesic, the primary action of which is based upon inhibition of prostaglandin synthesis (Majerus and Stanford, 1977). The superiority of diflunisal on the first post-operative day over codeine can likely be ascribed to this mechanism of action, as the concentration of prostaglandin is largest immediately in connection with the trauma, i.e. the surgical procedure (Holdcroft, 1975). It can be debated whether the oral dosage of codeine (25 mg q.i.d.) is sufficient to be analgesic in action, but most textbooks would accept this dosage as being reasonably analgesic (Goodman and Gilman, 1975). Increasing the codeine dosage would also lead to more adverse reactions from the gastroin-

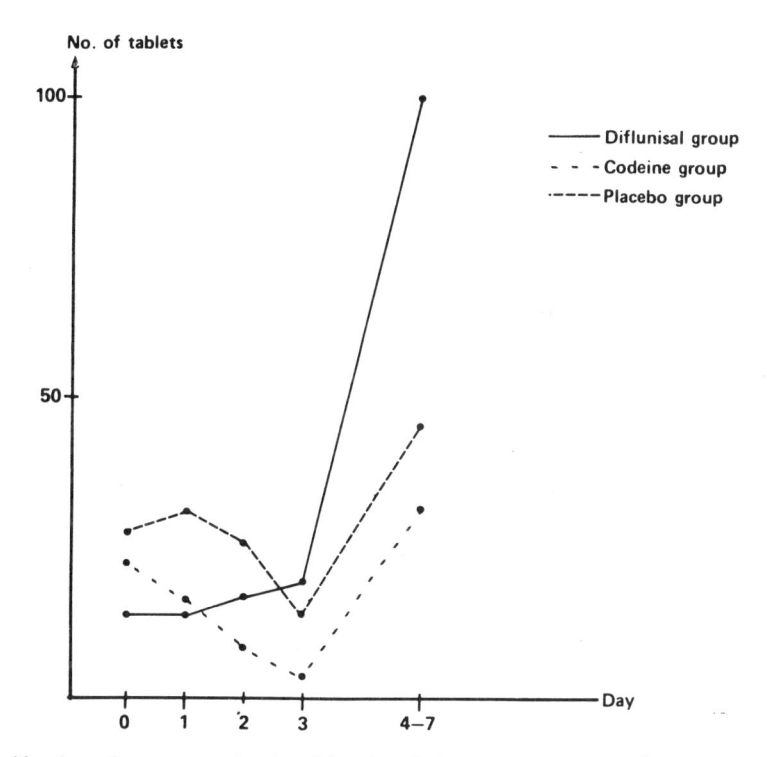

Figure 5. Number of reserve analgesic tablets in relation to test groups and post-operative days.

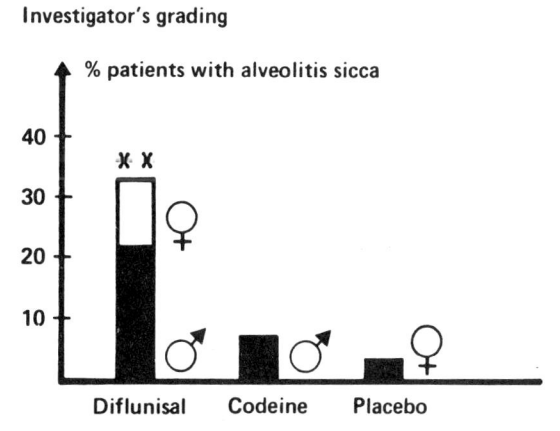

Figure 6. Bar diagram of number of patients with alveolitis sicca dolorosa (= "dry socket").
* *$P < 0.01$.

testinal tract, the incidence of which are already noticeable at the administered test dosage (Table 8). The constipating effect of codeine was lessened by adding 300 mg of Mg (OH)$_2$ to each 25 mg tablet of codeine phosphate.

The anti-inflammatory effect of diflunisal, that is the anti-swelling effect, is not pronounced (Figs 1 and 2) compared to that of codeine or lactose. The reason for this is probably due to the fact that post-operative swelling in this region is caused by inflammatory exudate, i.e. oedema, and interstitial bleeding, i.e. haematoma (Fig. 3). Sometimes, the haematoma can become quite large due to the loose structure of the tissues in this region. It is therefore important to minimize the risk of post-operative bleeding or oozing. Aspirin is a poor choice today as a post-operative analgesic for this reason (Hepsø et al., 1976).

Another facet of anti-inflammatory effect is the action of diflunisal on the muscles of mastication. Surgical procedures in the posterior region of the mandible tend to affect the medial or internal pterygoid muscle and the masseter muscle, both elevators or mouth-closing muscles of the mandible. Postoperatively, slight-oedema and inflammation in these muscles will result in decreased function. Clinically, this will appear as a diminished ability to open up maximally, a condition known as trismus. Diflunisal demonstrated a significantly better effect on trismus on day 1 than codeine or placebo (Fig. 3). This finding is most likely an anti-inflammatory effect.

There was no statistically significant difference in the incidence of adverse reaction among the three test groups, although the incidence is higher in the codeine group, as could be expected. The adverse reactions in the codeine group stem primarily from the central nervous system and the gastrointestinal tract.

One rather distressing finding, occurring on day 2–4 was the condition known as "dry socket" or alveolitis sicca dolorosa. In the diflunisal group, 10 out of 30 patients (33%) developed this most painful condition. In the codeine group only two patients and in the placebo group only one patient developed "dry socket". Therefore, the difference is highly statistically significant. "Dry socket" is caused by fibrinolysis of the blood clot in the alveolus (Birn, 1973). At the same time pain-inducing substances such as bradykinin and histamine are formed. This explains the rather high increase in consumption of reserve analgesic tablets after day 3 in the diflunisal group (Fig. 5). The data of the 10 patients with "dry socket" in the diflunisal group were carefully analysed for any possible causative factors but without success.

As diflunisal was administered before surgery, the forming blood clot in the alveolus after surgery would contain diflunisal in a measurable concentration, as the peak plasma level is reached in 2 h (Tempero et al., 1977). It is currently not known if diflunisal in some way will induce formation of plasmin from plasminogen, the fibrinolytic system. In another study by the author (Petersen, 1978), where the diflunisal was given post-operative as 500 mg t.i.d. using the same experimental model, the incidence of dry socket was 18% in the diflunisal group (5 out of 28 patients) versus 15% in the placebo group (4 out of 27 patients), a frequency which is in accordance with other studies (Birn, 1973). As the drug in the latter study was not taken until 3–4 h post-operatively, i.e. after the clot in the socket had formed and therefore could contain none or very little diflunisal, this seems to be the crucial point. More studies should be done to elucidate this intriguing problem.

Conclusion

Diflunisal 500 mg b.i.d. demonstrates a statistically significantly better analgesic effect on day 1 post-operatively following surgical removal of impacted third molars than does codeine phosphate 25 mg q.i.d. and lactose as placebo. On day 3 post-operatively, the differences are not statistically significantly different. Diflunisal will also reduce trismus more on day 1 post-operatively than codeine and placebo. There is currently no explanation for an observed high and significant increase in the post-operative complication known as "dry socket" in the diflunisal group.

References

Birn, H. (1973). *Int. J. Oral Surg.* 2, 211–267.
Goodman, L. S. and Gilman, A. (1975). "The Pharmacological Basis of Therapeutics", 5th ed., p. 256, Macmillan Publishing Company Inc., New York.
Hepsø, H. V., Løkken, P., Bjørson, J., and Godal, H. C. (1976). *Eur. J. Clin. Pharmac.* 10, 217–225.
Holdcroft, A. (1975). *Anaesth. Intern. Case.* 3, 105–113.
Majerus, P. W. and Stanford, N. (1977). *Brit. J. Clin. Pharmac.* 4, 15–18 (Suppl. 1).
Moroz, L. A. (1977). *New Eng. J. Med.* 296, 525–529.
Petersen, J. K. (1975). *Int. J. Oral Surg.* 4, 267–276.
Petersen, J. K. (1978). *Int. J. Oral Surg.* (In press).
Smit-Sibinga, C. Th. (1977). *Brit. J. Clin. Pharmac.* 4, 375–385.
Temporo, K. F., Cirillo, V. J., and Steelman, S. L. (1977). *Brit. J. Clin. Pharmac.* 4, 31–36 (Suppl. 1).

Summary

In a double-blind, randomized study of the analgesic and anti-inflammatory efficacy of diflunisal 500 mg b.i.d. versus codeine phosphate 25 mg q.i.d., versus placebo in pain and swelling following surgical removal of impacted third molars, diflunisal was found to be superior to codeine and placebo on the first post-operative day. The difference in efficacy of the drugs diminished on the third post-operative day. In the diflunisal group of 30 patients, 10 of them (33%) developed "dry socket" or alveolitis sicca dolorosa. Only two patients in the codeine group and one patient in the placebo group developed this very painful condition. The possible explanation of "dry socket" is discussed.

Zusammenfassung

In einer doppelt blinden, wahllosen Studie der analgesischen und entzündungsverhütenden Wirksamkeit von Diflunisal 500 mg zweimal täglich gegen Kodeinphosphat 25 mg viermal täglich gegen Placebo im Schmerz und in der Schwellung nach einer chirurgischen Entfernung von eingekeilten Weisheitszähnen erwies sich Diflunisal am ersten Tag nach der Operation als Kodein und Placebo überlegen. Der Unterschied in der Wirksamkeit der Drogen wurde am dritten Tag nach der Operation geringer. In der Diflunisal-Gruppe von 30 Patienten entwickelten 10 von ihnen (33%) ein "trockenes Zahnfach" oder Alveolitis Sicca Dolorosa. Nur zwei Patienten in der Kodein-Gruppe und ein Patient in der Placebo-Gruppe entwickelten diesen äußerst schmerzhaften Zustand. Die mögliche Erklärung für das "trockene Zahnfach" wird erörtert.

Résumé

Dans une étude aléatorisée à double anonymat sur l'efficacité analgésique et anti-inflammatoire du diflunisal (2×500 mg par jour) et du phosphate de codéine (4×25 mg par jour) par comparaison avec un placebo contre la douleur et l'enflure à la suite de l'extraction de troisièmes molaires encastrées, on constate que le diflunisal est supérieur à la codéine et au placebo le premier jour après l'opération. La différence d'efficacité des deux médicaments diminue le troisième jour après l'opération. Dans le groupe "diflunisal" de 30 sujets, 10 (33%) présentent une alvéolite sèche douloureuse. Deux sujets seulement du groupe "codéine" et un seul du groupe "placebo" présentent cette affection très douloureuse. On propose une explication possible de l'alvéolite sèche douloureuse.

Sommario

In uno studio casualizzato e "double-blind" dell'efficacia analgesica e antiflogistica del diflunisal (500 mg due volte al giorno) a raffronto del fosfato di codeina (25 mg 4 volte al giorno) nochè di placebo (sostanza innocua somministrata a scopo di controllo), in presenza di dolori e gonfiori seguenti l'asportazione chirurgica di denti del giudizio incuneati, si trovò il diflunisal superiore alla codeina e placebo nel primo giorno dopo l'operazione. La differenza nell'efficacia dei medicamenti diminuisce nel terzo giorno dopo l'operazione. In 10 dei 30 pazienti costituenti il gruppo diflunisal (pari al 33%) si manifestò un'alveolite secca, a raffronto di solo 2 pazienti del gruppo codeina e di un solo paziente nel gruppo placebo. Si discutono le cause probabili di tale alveolite secca.

Resumen

En un estudio aleatorio a doble ciego acerca de la eficacia analgésica y antinflamatoria del diflunisal en dosis de 500 mg dos veces al día, comparado con fosfato de codeína de 25 mg 4 veces al día y un placebo sobre el dolor y la hinchazón tras la extracción quirúrgica de terceros molares impactados, se comprobó que el diflunisal es superior a la codeína y al placebo en el primer día después de la operación. La diferencia de eficacia entre los medicamentos disminuyó al tercer día de la operación. De los 30 pacientes del grupo del diflunisal, 10 (33%) desarrollaron una alveolitis seca dolorosa. Sólo dos pacientes en el grupo de la codeína y uno en el de placebo desarrollaron esta condición dolorosa. Se analiza aquí la posible explicación de la alveolitis.

Sumário

Num estudo, duplamente às cegas e ao acaso, sobre a eficácia analgésica e anti-inflamatória do diflunisal (500 mg duas vezes por dia) em comparação com o fosfato de codeína (25 mg quatro vezes por dia), e ainda com um placebo, no alívio de dor e inchaço em seguida à extracção cirúrgica de três dentes molares encravados, o diflunisal provou ser superior à codeína e placebo no primeiro dia post-operatório.

A diferença no grau de eficácia das drogas diminuiu no terceiro dia post-operatório. No grupo diflunisal formado por 30 doentes, 10 deles (33%) desenvolveram alveolite sêca dolorosa. Apenas dois doentes do grupo codeína e um doente do grupo placebo desenvolveram esta complicação que é extremamente dolorosa. A possível explicação da ocorrência de "alvéolo sêco" é discutida no relatório.

Analgesic Effect of Diflunisal in Perineorrhaphy

S. PEIXOTO, M. B. SANTINHO and C. A. SALVATORE

Gynaecology Clinic of University of Sao Paulo, Medical School, Sao Paulo, Brazil

---

Perineorrhaphy is mandatory in most vaginal surgical procedures to correct perineal ruptures frequently associated with the underlying primary pathology. In addition to this, perineorrhaphy, by approximating components of the elevator muscle of the anus, provides strengthening of the perineal base and of the genital supporting structures.

From a technical point of view, the different layers sutured have to be considered as a whole with the muscular structures involved, in particular the "local traumatic area" including vascular and nervous tissues. Superficial vascular formations call for local haemostasia with successive suture stitches which involve, in variable proportions, compression of peri-vascular tissues. During surgery local tissue damage or tension of tissue edges and post-operative haemostasia, while preventing local haemorrhages, frequently leads to local discomfort and contributes an additional cause of local pain. Local pain due to surgical incision is therefore more evident in the post-operative period.

The object of this study was to evaluate the reduction of pain at the perineorrhaphy scar site, following prophylactic administration of a new analgesic compound, diflunisal.

Materials and Methods

Diflunisal is a derivative of salicyclic acid launched in 1971 for clinical trial as an anti-inflammatory agent. In the present study it was used orally in 125 mg tablets but it is also available in 250 and 500 mg tablets to allow dosage variations.

The trial covered a total of 39 patients who had vaginal surgery and in whom pain in the scar of the perineorrhaphy could be assessed. The patients were divided into three groups:
 1. 19 patients treated with diflunisal;
 2. 12 patients treated with a similar analgesic agent, Doloxene-A, (propoxyphene napsylate, 100 mg and acetylsalicylic acid 325 mg);

3. 8 patients receiving no analgesic therapy (control group).

The three groups were similar in terms of age, height and weight and the type of surgery was comparable (Table 1).

Table 1

Type of surgery performed

Type of surgery	Groups		
	I	II	III
Colpoperineorrhaphy	11	4	8
"Manchester"	4	5	–
Vaginal hysterectomy	4	3	–

The patients in groups 1 and 2 were given the analgesic agent during the first 24 h after surgery, according to the following schedule:

Diflunisal—500 mg by oral route every 12 h

Comparative drug—one capsule by oral route every 6 h.

It was accepted that pain was related to both objective and subjective factors and it was assessed in terms of inflammation, infection and trauma associated with the sutures and local compression of the vagina. On the other hand, secondary effects such as intestinal motility, lung ventilation and thromboembolism were also assessed.

The effect of diflunisal was assessed during all the surgical prodecures, beginning in the pre-operative period with a clinical and laboratory evaluation including haemoglobin, creatinine, bilirubin, SGOT and alkaline phosphatase. These variables were evaluated again in the post-operative phase, i.e. 3–10 days after surgery. The assessment was based on the local aspect of the surgical wound, continued maintenance of vesical drainage, sufficient vaginal tamponment and evaluation of emotional state. The possible systemic effects of the drug were assessed by clinical tolerance and analysis of the post-operative laboratory data.

Results

Local pain was reported during the first post-operative day as follows:
  Group 1 (diflunisal)—3/19 (15·78%)
  Group 2 (Doloxene-A)—3/12 (25%)
  Group 3 (control)—6/8 (75%)

With regard to comparative therapeutic activity, effective analgesia was present in 16/19 patients receiving diflunisal (84·2%) and in 9/12 receiving Doloxene-A (75%).

Drug tolerance was good since no allergic nor gastrointestinal disorders were reported.

The systemic effect of the drug before and after surgery is shown in Table 2.

Table 2

Laboratory Parameters	Mean Values	
	Pre	Post
Haemoglobin (g%)	13·08	12·46
Creatinine (mg%)	0·89	0·91
Total bilirubin (mg%)	0·58	0·57
SGOT (units/ml)	11·70	13·31
Alkaline phosphatase (units)	105·94	101·98

In all groups there was no evidence of leukocytosis, either in the pre- or post-surgery evaluations which reduces the possibility of secondary contamination of the wound, and consequent local discomfort.

Discussion

Pain in surgical scars has motivated continual research into analgesic compounds not only to provide physical and psychic comfort to the patient but also to prevent post-operative complications such as immobility, venous stasis, soft tissue compression associated with respiratory disturbances and eventually pulmonary insufficiency (Moore, 1971).

Available therapy includes compounds at the extremes of clinical efficacy. Van Winzum and Rodda (1977) stressed the risks of injectable analgesics as well as the poor activity of oral analgesics, based on post-surgical observations.

Local pain in a surgical scar is associated with many factors. Faintuch (1978) showed the importance of the substrate phase, extending to the fourth day post-surgery, with problems of local vascularization, clotting and trauma. Depending on the extent of the devitalized area, local coagulation and bacterial colonization with different degrees of pain are also evident. These factors are usually present most intensely in the 24 h following surgery and in the case of perineorrhaphy they are markedly present. In our population, pain was spontaneously evident in 75% of the control group.

Pain consequent to vaginal surgery is referred at the surgical scar site due to trauma of the surrounding structures. Urethral involvement is frequent, mainly subsequent to catheterization during surgery or following operation to maintain vesical drainage. Urethral sensitivity to micro-organisms can produce local discomfort without clinical evidence of urinary infection and analgesics with a high urinary excretion could, to a certain extent, relieve some of the factors contributing to pain. Tempero et al. (1977) evaluated urinary elimination of diflunisal measuring excretion of prostaglandin metabolites E_1 and E_2. Their findings were a 70% reduction of these metabolites 12 h after drug intake, confirming results of Steelman et al. (1976). In the present study, evaluated solely by clinical manifestation of pain, efficacy was evident as early as 8 h after medication. Our observations are supported by experimental data of Tocco et al. (1975) showing maximum plasma reactivity levels 2h after oral administration of 50 or 500 mg of diflunisal.

Diflunisal is a 5-(2-4 difluorophenyl)salicylic derivative which does not act by acetylating proteins and macromolecules (Hannah et al., 1977; Shen 1977). This pharmacodynamic modification produces better analgesic potency and longer duration of action (Maierus and Stanford, 1977). In our population this aspect was evaluated comparing the effect of diflunisal with a similar analgesic combination product: diflunisal administered at 12 h intervals produced analgesic efficacy in 84·22% of patients compared to 75% of the combination administered at 6-h intervals.

The relation of local pain to surgical technique should be emphasized. Extension of the devitalized area, local tension conditions and so on, should be considered, together with the materials used for the surgical reconstruction. Livingstone et al. (1974) pointed out the lower degree of local pain when using a thread made of polyglycolic material. In the present study, the material used was catgut which generally lessens local pain. As it is a common denominator for all material, its use did not change the results but permitted an accurate evaluation of the potency of the test drug.

Although diflunisal and ASA present similar anti-inflammatory analgesic and antipyretic properties, their gastric effects are of a different degree. Stone et al. (1977) indicated that both drugs had a tendency to cause gastric irritation, based on experimental data. In our population, no evidence of this was found.

Conclusions

1. Pain is a common manifestation in the post-operative period of vaginal surgery. Without using any prophylactic medication, clinically, its frequency in our population was of 75%.
2. With the prophylactic administration of diflunisal, pain was reported in 15·78% of patients.
3. The analgesic effect occurs probably 2 h after intake.
4. No intolerance to diflunisal was seen by clinical evaluation of the cases.
5. No systemic effect of the drug was evident prior to surgery and 3–10 days in the post-operative period.

References

Faintuch, J., Machado, M. C. C. and Raia, A. (1978). "Manual de pre e pos operatorio." Editora Manole Ltda. Sao Paulo.
Hannah, W. V. R., Jones, H., Kelly, K. W., Witzel, B. E., Holtz, W. J., Houser, R. W., Shen, T. Y., and Sarett, L. H. (1977). "The Discovery of Diflunisal". Merck Sharpe & Dohme Research Laboratories, Rahway, New Jersey, USA.
Majerus, P. W. and Stanford, N. (1977). "Comparative Effects of Aspirin and Diflunisal on Prostaglandin Synthetase from Human and Sheep Seminal vesicles". National Institute of Health Specialized Centre for Research in Thrombosis.
Moore, F. D. (1971). "Critical Surgical Illness". W. B. Saunders Company, Philadelphia, USA.
Shen, T. Y. (1977). "The Discovery of Diflunisal", Merck Sharpe & Dohme Research Laboratories, West Point, Pennsylvania, USA.
Stone, C. A. et al. (1977). "Pharmacology and Toxicology of Diflunisal", Merck Sharpe & Dohme Research Laboratories, West Point, Pennsylvania, USA.

Tempero, K. F., Cirillo, V. J. and Steelman, S. L. (1977). *Brit. J. Clin. Pharmac.* **4,** 31.
Tocco, D. J., Breault, G. O., Zacchei, A. G., Steelman, S. L. and Perrier, C. V. (1975). *Drug Met. Dis.* **3,** 453.
Van Winzum, C. and Rodda, B. (1977). "Diflunisal: Efficacy in Post-operative Pain", Merck Sharpe & Dohme Research Laboratories, Rahway, New Jersey, USA.
Livingstone, E., Simpson, D. and Naismith, W. C. M. K. (1974). *J. Obstet. Gynaecol. Brit. Commonwealth* **81,** 245.

Summary

Thirty-nine patients who had undergone vaginal surgery were given either diflunisal (500 mg every 12 h), Doloxene-A (one capsule every 6 h) or no treatment, in the 24 h immediately post-operation. Local pain was reported in 16% of patients taking diflunisal, in 25% taking Doloxene-A and in 75% of controls. The analgesic effect of diflunisal appeared to occur 2 h after ingestion of the drug and no intolerance to it was noted.

Zusammenfassung

Neununddreißig Patienten, an denen ein vaginaler chirurgischer Eingriff vorgenommen worden war, wurde entweder Diflunisal (500 mg alle 12 Stunden), Doloxene-A (eine Kapsel alle sechs Stunden) verabreicht bzw. sie erhielten keinerlei Behandlung innerhalb der 24 Stunden unmittelbar nach der Operation. Örtlicher Schmerz wurde in 16% der Diflunisal einnehmenden Patienten festgestellt, in 25% der Doloxene-A einnehmenden Patienten, und in 75% der Kontrollpersonen. Die analgesische Wirkung von Diflunisal schien zwei Stunden nach Einnehmen der Droge aufzutreten, und es wurde keine Unverträglichkeit festgestellt.

Résumé

Trente-neuf malades ayant subi des opérations du vagin reçoivent soit 500 mg de diflunisal toutes les 12 heures, soit une capsule de Doloxène-A toutes les six heures, soit aucun traitement, pendant 24 heures après l'opération. Des douleurs locales sont notées chez 16% des malades recevant du diflunisal, 25% des malades recevant du Doloxène-A et 75% des malades témoins. L'effet analgésique du diflunisal paraît se produire deux heures après ingestion; on ne note aucune intolérance.

Sommario

Durante le 24 ore seguenti l'intervento chirurgico vaginale, a 39 pazienti venne somministrato il diflunisal (500 mg ogni 12 ore) oppure Doloxene-A (una capsula ogni sei ore) ovvero nulla del tutto. Rispettivamente il 16%, 25% e 75% dei pazienti dei gruppi diflunisal, Doloxene-A e di controllo denunciarono algie localizzate. L'effetto analgesico del diflunisal apparve verificarsi due ore dopo l'ingestione del medicamento e non si notò alcuna intolleranza.

Resumen

Treinta y nueve pacientes que habían tenido operaciones vaginales recibieron ya sea diflunisal (500 mg cada 12 horas), Doloxene-A (un comprimido cada 6 horas) o ningún tratamiento en las primeras 24 horas después de la operación. Se comprobó que el 16% de los pacientes con diflunisal tuvieron dolor localizado en comparación con el 25% con Doloxene-A y el 75% en los testigos. El efecto analgésico del diflunisal pareció producirse a las dos horas de tomar el medicamento y no se observó intolerancia.

Sumário

Trinta e nove doentes que tinham sido submetidas a cirurgia vaginal, receberam diflunisal (500 mg de 12 em 12 horas), ou Doloxene-A (uma cápsula de seis em seis horas), ou nenhum tratamento, nas 24 horas imediatamente depois da operação. Queixas de dor local foram feitas por 16% das doentes que tomaram diflunisal, 25% das que tomaram Doloxene-A, e 75% das testemunhas. O efeito analgésico do diflunisal parecia ocorrer duas horas após ingestão da droga, e não se observaram quaisquer sinais de intolerância.

Diflunisal compared with Pentazocine in the Relief of Pain following Knee Surgery

D. GOUTALLIER and J. DEBEYRE

*Department of Orthopaedic Surgery,
Henri Mondor, Creteil, France*

Pain following surgery is less intense after the first 48 h and the dose of any analgesic such as diflunisal ought to be high up to that point and then lowered in the following post-operative period. In this study such a regime was used and compared to the effect of a fixed dosage of pentazocine which is a potent analgesic with an effective duration of action of 6 h.

Materials and Methods

Forty patients aged between 19 and 71 years, and who complained of moderate to severe pain in the morning following knee surgery, were selected. Short acting analgesics were permitted on the day of surgery but no analgesics or anti-inflammatory agents were given from 4 h prior to the first test dose until 6 h after the last. The study was double-blind and the patients were randomized into two groups.
    (1) Diflunisal: Day 1 and 2—500 mg b.i.d.
                      Day 3, 4 and 5—250 mg b.i.d.
    (2) Pentazocine: 50 mg q.i.d. throughout all days.
    The patients in the diflunisal group received placebo tablets between each active dose so that both groups were taking tablets every 6 h.
    Spontaneous pain was recorded each morning and evening on a 4-point scale (0 = no pain; 1 = mild, intermittent but not interfering with sleep; 2 = constant, moderate pain but allowing sleep; 4 = severe). Tenderness was also recorded in the morning only, again on a 4-point scale (0 = no pain on firm pressure; 1 = mild pain on firm pressure; 2 = mild to moderate pain on firm pressure, 3 = severe pain on gentle pressure). On days 2 to 5 the patients evaluated the efficacy of the test therapy and the investigator did so at the conclusion of the study, both using the same rating scale. On the morning of day 1, before the first medication, all patients in the diflunisal group (20) had severe pain and in the pentazocine group, 18 had severe and 2 moderate pain.
    The two treatment groups were similar in regard to weight, sex, surgical procedure and importance of trauma (Table 1). However, the mean ages of the diflunisal group and pentazocine group differed significantly (Table 2).

Diflusinal: Royal Society of Medicine International Congress and Symposium Series No. 6, published jointly by Academic Press Inc. (London) Ltd., and the Royal Society of Medicine.

Table 1

Knee surgery

	Diflunisal			Pentazocine		
Importance of surgical trauma	Mild	Moderate	Severe	Mild	Moderate	Severe
Tibial osteotomy	—	3	3	—	2	—
Femoral osteotomy	—	—	1	—	—	—
Menisectomy	1	1	—	—	1	1
Fracture plateau tibiae	—	1	1	—	—	—
Transposition tuberositas tibiae	—	3	1	—	8	1
Foreign body removal	—	2	—	—	2	—
Arthrotomy	—	—	—	1	—	—
Lindeman[a]	—	—	3	—	—	2
Repair of sprain[a]	—	—	—	—	—	2
TOTAL =	1	10	9	1	13	6

[a] Patients with plaster cast.

Table 2

Age (years)

	Diflunisal	Pentazocine
Mean	48·4	36·3[a]
Medium	51·0	28·0
Range	19–71	19–64

[a] Statistically significant differences $P < 0.05$.

Results

Four patients on diflunisal and six on pentazocine discontinued the treatment due to ineffective therapy. These patients were considered to be treatment failures. One patient on diflunisal discontinued on day 4 due to pulmonary embolism which was not drug related.

Eight patients on diflunisal and six on pentazocine had mild or no spontaneous pain on the evening of day 1, and on the morning of day 3 there were 16 such patients on diflunisal and 12 patients on pentazocine (Fig. 1). There were no statistically significant differences between the two groups. Figure 2 shows the mean tenderness curves of the two treatment groups which follow each other very closely.

Table 3 indicates the patient's assessment of the efficacy of the test therapy and Table 4 the investigator's opinion. It is clear that the results are similar in the two groups.

Clinical tolerance of both drugs was good and only four patients in both groups had slight drug-related side-effects, mainly gastrointestinal upset or headache.

No data are available on the biological tolerance in this study because laboratory tests were performed only at the entry of the study.

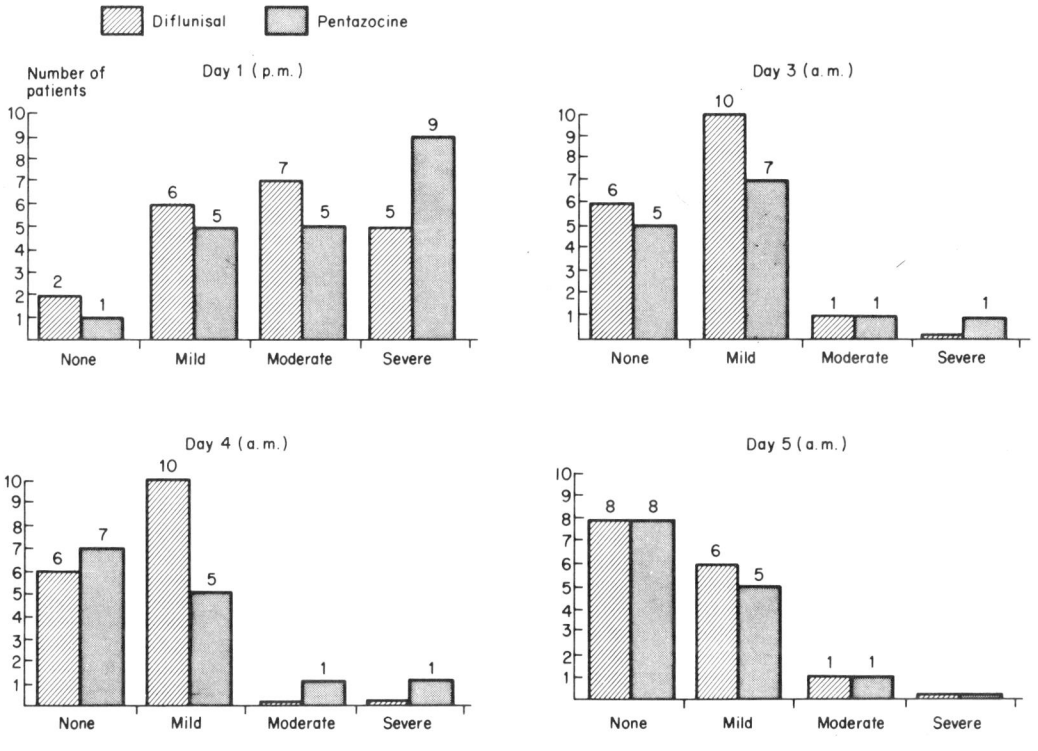

Figure 1. Relief of spontaneous pain.

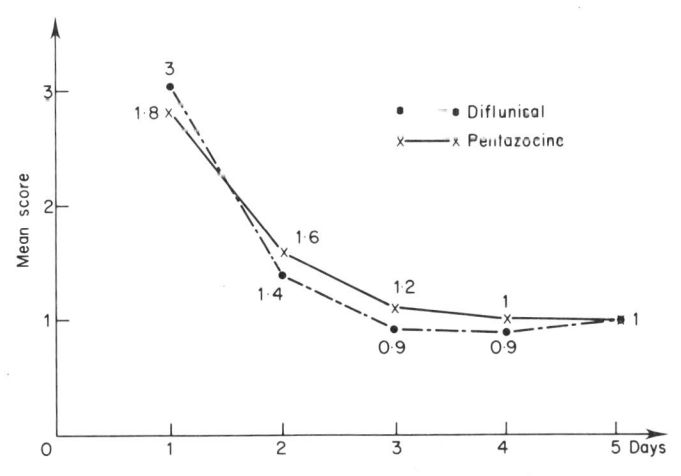

Figure 2. Effect of diflunisal and pentazocine on tenderness scores.

Table 3

Patient's assessment

Evaluation	Treatment group	Good	Fair	Poor	None	Drop out[a]	Total
Day 2	Diflunisal	10	4	3	1	2	20
	Pentazocine	8	2	3	3	3	19[b]
Day 3	Diflunisal	13	4	—	—	3	20
	Pentazocine	9	2	2	1	6	20
Day 4	Diflunisal	13	3	—	—	4	20
	Pentazocine	11	1	1	1	6	20
Day 5	Diflunisal	13	2	—	—	4	19[c]
	Pentazocine	11	1	1	1	6	20

[a] Due to ineffective therapy.
[b] One patient did not assess treatment.
[c] One patient had a pulmonary embolism and was removed from the study on Day 4.
There were no statistically significant differences between the treatment groups.

Table 4

Investigator's opinion

Investigator's evaluation	Excellent	Fair	Poor	None
Diflunisal (20)	12	4	2	2
Pentazocine (20)	8	4	6	2

Conclusion

In this double-blind randomized study, 40 patients with moderate or severe postoperative pain were allocated to either diflunisal or pentazocine group. Diflunisal 500 mg b.i.d. is as active as pentazocine 50 q.i.d. in the relief of pain following knee surgery in the first two days and diflunisal, 250 mg b.i.d., is equal to pentazocine 50 q.i.d. in the treatment of pain on days 3 to 5.

Summary

The purpose of the trial was to study the efficacy and safety of diflunisal and pentazocine in the relief of pain following knee surgery: 40 patients with moderate to severe pain were randomized in two groups. Diflunisal dosage was 500 mg b.i.d. for the first 2 days, then diflunisal 250 mg b.i.d. or pentazocine 50 mg q.i.d. during 5 days in double-blind. The treatment groups were similar with regard to pretreatment characteristics except for the mean age (36·3 years in pentazocine and 48·4 in diflunisal). Spontaneous pain, tenderness, patient and investigator openions were recorded.

Results were evaluated as excellent or good in 12 of the 20 (60%) patients on diflunisal, and eight of the 20 (40%) patients on pentazocine. Four patients on diflunisal and six on pentazocine had unbearable pain and needed other analgesics. No statistically significant differences between groups were found. Tolerance was excellent, except in four patients on diflunisal and four on pentazocine who reported some drug-related adverse reactions.

Zusammenfassung

Zweck des Versuches war das Studium der Wirksamkeit und Sicherheit von Diflunisal und Pentazocin in der Linderung von Schmerz nach einem Eingriff im Knie. Vierzig Patienten mit mäßigem bis heftigem Schmerz wurden wahllos in zwei Gruppen aufgeteilt. Die Diflunisal-Dosis betrug 500 mg zweimal täglich während der ersten beiden Tage, sodann Diflunisal 250 mg zweimal täglich, und die Pentazocin-Dosierung betrug 50 mg viermal täglich während der Dauer von fünf Tagen in einem doppelt blinden Versuch. Die Behandlungsgruppen waren in bezug auf Vorbehandlungscharakteristiken ähnlich, ausgenommen das mittlere Alter (36,3 Jahre in Pentazocin und 48,4 in Diflunisal). Spontanschmerz, Weichheit, Patienten- und Untersucher-Meinungen wurden vermerkt.

Die Ergebnisse wurden als ausgezeichnet oder gut in 12 der 20 (60%) Patienten auf Diflunisal, und 8 von den 20 (40%) Patienten auf Pentazocin ausgewertet. Vier Patienten auf Diflunisal und 6 auf Pentazocine hatten unerträgliche Schmerzen und benötigten andere schmerzlindernde Mittel. Es wurden keine statistisch bedeutsamen Unterschiede zwischen den Gruppen festgestellt. Die Verträglichkeit war ausgezeichnet, mit Ausnahme von 5 Patienten auf Diflunisal und 4 auf Pentazocin, die einige widrige Reaktionen meldeten.

Résumé

Le but de l'essai est d'étudier l'efficacité et l'innocuité du diflunisal et de la pentazocine sur le soulagement de la douleur après une opération du genou. Quarante malades souffrant de douleurs modérées à aiguës sont répartis au hasard en deux groupes. La posologie du diflunisal est de 2 × 500 mg par jour les deux premiers jours, puis 250 mg par jour; la posologie de la pentazocine est de 4 × 50 mg par jour pendant cinq jours, en double anonymat. Les deux groupes se ressemblent beaucoup au point de vue des caractéristiques avant traitement, sauf pour l'âge moyen (36,5 ans dans le groupe "pentazocine", 48,4 ans dans le groupe "diflunisal"). On note la douleur spontanée, la sensibilité, et les opinions du malade et de l'observateur.

Les résultats sont notés "excellents" ou "bons" pour 12 des 20 malades du groupe "diflunisal" (60%) et 8 des 20 malades du groupe "pentazocine" (40%). Quatre malades du groupe "diflunisal" et six malades du groupe "pentazocine", souffrant de douleurs intolérables, ont dû recevoir d'autres analgésiques. On ne constate aucune différence significative entre les deux groupes. La tolérance est excellente, sauf pour 5 malades du groupe "diflunisal" et 4 malades du groupe "pentazocine", qui présentaient des réactions défavorables.

Sommario

La prova ha avuto come scopo lo studio dell'efficacia e sicurezza del diflunisal e pentazocina nel trattamento del dolore in seguito ad intervento chirurgico al ginocchio. Si suddivisero a caso in due gruppi 40 pazienti con dolori da lievi a intensi. Il diflunisal venne somministrato in dosi di 500 mg due volte al giorno per i primi due giorni e quindi in dosi di 250 mg due volte al giorno, mentre la pentazocina in dosi di 50 mg 4 volte al giorno per i 5 giorni della prova, secondo il metodo "double-blind".
I gruppi erano simili per quanto riguardava le caratteristiche di pretrattamento eccetto per l'età media (36,3 anni nel pentazocine e 48,4 nel diflunisal). Si prese nota del dolore spontaneo e al tatto, nonchè delle opinioni del paziente e dei ricercatori.
I risultati furono stimati eccellenti oppure buoni in 12 dei 20 (60%) pazienti del gruppo diflunisal, e in 8 dei 20 (40%) pazienti del gruppo pentazocina. Quattro pazienti del gruppo diflunisal e 6 del gruppo pentazocina presentarono dolori insostenibili e si dovette loro somministrare altri analgesici. Non si trovò alcuna differenza statisticamente significativa tra i due gruppi. La tolleranza fu eccellente eccetto per 5 pazienti del gruppo diflunisal e 4 del gruppo pentazocina, i quali dichiararono alcune reazioni avverse.

Resumen

El propósito de este estudio fue estudiar la eficacia y seguridad del diflunisal y la pentazocina en el alivio del dolor luego de cirugía de rodilla. Se dividieron al azar 40 pacientes en dos grupos. La dosis de diflunisal fue de 500 mg dos veces por día en los primeros días y luego 250 mg dos veces por día, y la de pentazocina 50 mg cuatro veces por día durante 5 días a doble ciego. Los dos grupos de pacientes eran semejantes respecto a ciertos riesgos previos al tratamiento, excepto en la edad media (36,3 años para pentazocina y 48,4 para diflunisal). Se tomó nota del dolor espontáneo y a la palpación y de las opiniones del paciente y el investigador.
Se obtuvieron resultados que se consideraron excelentes o buenos en 12 de los 20 pacientes (60%) sometidos a diflunisal y 8 de los 20 (40%) a pentazocina. Cuatro pacientes con diflunisal y 6 con pentazocina experimentaron dolores intolerables que necesitaron otros analgésicos. No se encontró diferencia estadística considerable entre los grupos. La tolerancia fue excelente excepto en 5 pacientes con diflunisal y 4 con pentazocina que manifestaron algunas reacciones adversas.

Sumário

O objectivo do ensaio era estudar a eficácia e grau de segurança do diflunisal e da pentazocina no alívio da dor após cirurgia no joelho. Quarenta doentes com dores moderadas a severas foram distribuídos ao acaso em dois grupos. A dose de diflunisal foi de 500 mg (2 vezes/dia) nos primeiros dois dias, seguida por 250 mg (2 vezes/dia); a dose de pentazocina foi de 50 mg (4 vezes/dia) durante cinco dias, num sistema às duplas cegas. Os grupos de tratamento eram idênticos quanto às características prétratamento, salvo no que dizia respeito à idade média (36,3 anos no grupo pentazocina e 48,4 anos no grupo diflunisal). Os parâmetros registados foram a dor espontânea, a sensibilidade à palpação, a opinião do doente e as opiniões dos investigadores.

Os resultados foram avaliados como excelentes ou bons em 12 (60%) dos 20 doentes do grupo diflunisal, e em 8 (40%) dos 20 doentes do grupo pentazocina. Quatro doentes do grupo diflunisal e 6 doentes do grupo pentazocina queixaram-se de dor intensa e insuportável, que requeriu outros analgésicos. Não se notaram quaisquer diferenças estatìsticamente significativas entre os dois grupos. A tolerância foi excelente, excepto em 5 doentes do grupo diflunisal e 4 do grupo pentazocina que se queixaram de algumas reacções adversas.

Diflunisal compared with Glafenine in Pain associated with Carcinoma

J. CHRISTODOULOPOULOS and E. HOUSSIANAKOU

*Metaxas Memorial Hospital for Cancer
Piraeus, Greece*

Analgesia is very often the major therapeutic help which can be offered to patients with carcinoma, so that any new analgesic agent is of potential interest to doctors dealing with such patients. The purpose of this study was to assess the analgesic activity of a new agent (diflunisal) and to compare it to glafenine, in patients with moderate and severe pain associated with various types of neoplastic diseases.

Materials and Methods

Patients with moderate or severe pain due to neoplastic disease were included in the study (Table 1). The patients were randomly allocated to two treatment groups; 19 received diflunisal and 17 glafenine.

The study was designed as single-blind and single-dose and prior to taking the test medication the patient recorded the intensity of spontaneous pain, which was scored as 0 for no pain, 1 = mild, 2 = moderate and 3 = severe. After a single dose of 500 mg of diflunisal (two 250 mg tablets), the intensity of the patient's pain was followed up and recorded at 1, 2, 4, 6, 8 and 10 h by the same investigator throughout the study (Dr E.H.). The score of pain relief was marked on a visual analogue scale reading from 0 = no relief at one end to 10 — complete relief at the other end. No other analgesic was allowed for at least 4 h before or during the study and if additional analgesia became necessary that patient was considered as having withdrawn from the study.

Results

Out of 36 patients who entered the study, 33 completed the trial according to the protocol. Two of the three who dropped out belonged to the glafenine group and were

Table 1

Type of cancer in trial patients

Diflunisal group					Glafenine group			
Patient	Sex	Age	Type of cancer		Patient	Sex	Age	Type of cancer
K.D.	F	75	Stomach cancer		P.J.	M	58	Stomach cancer
N.A.	F	60	Breast cancer		Z.G.	M	36	Lung cancer
H.G.	M	50	Metastatic bone cancer		P.G.	M	60	Acute leukemia
Z.C.	F	53	Breast cancer		L.E.	F	40	Acute leukemia
M.E.	F	60	Breast cancer		D.S.	M	65	Leukemia
M.N.	M	33	Acute leukemia		S.P.	M	60	Lymphoma
M.A.	M	65	Acute leukemia		R.P.	M	55	Lymphoma
B.E.	F	43	Liver cancer		G.P.	F	72	Stomach cancer
P.E.	M	57	Multiple myeloma		K.A.	F	68	Multiple myeloma
S.D.	F	69	Multiple myeloma		V.P.	M	53	Lung cancer
V.A.	M	61	Lung cancer		N.A.	F	56	Breast cancer
P.E.	F	50	Breast cancer		P.M.	F	59	Breast cancer
R.M.	F	72	Multiple myeloma		M.L.	M	68	Multiple myeloma
A.N.	M	55	Lymphoma		G.A.	M	44	Lymphoma
B.G.	M	48	Lung cancer		P.G.	F	50	Breast cancer
M.A.	F	47	Breast cancer		I.A.	M	58	Lung cancer
F.A.	M	38	Lymphoma					
A.V.	M	56	Lung cancer					

Table 2

Time of assesment (h)	Intensity of spontaneous pain									
	Diflunisal					Glafenine				
	0	1	2	3	Total*	0	1	2	3	Total*
Pre-treatment	0	0	9	9	18	0	0	6	9	15
1	6	6	5	1	18	5	7	2	1	15
2	12	3	2	1	18	9	4	1	1	15
4	11	3	3	1	18	9	2	1	3	15
6	11	1	3	3	18	8	2	0	5	15
8	11	0	3	4	18	8	1	0	6	15
10	11	0	3	4	18	8	0	1	6	15

Scale: 0 = no pain; 1 = mild pain; 2 = moderate; 3 = severe.
*Number of patients.

not evaluated because both vomited 10 min after the administration of the drug. The third patient who was taking diflunisal, was considered as a drop-out on the grounds that he experienced withdrawal symptoms after being taken off his routine analgesic treatment with dextropropoxyphene.

In the 33 patients who completed the study both drugs have shown significant analgesic activity (Table 2). When the Wilcoxon rank sum test was employed no significant difference was found between pain grade 0, 1, 2, and 3 of patients treated with diflunisal or glafenine. Figure 1 shows, in graphic form, the evolution of the pain intensity during the observation time.

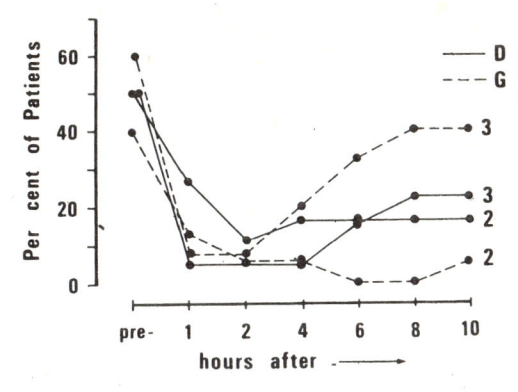

Figure 1. Evolution of pain intensity.

Conclusions

The presented data show clearly that both drugs exhibited significant analgesic activity and can control the moderate and severe pain caused by carcinoma, in a considerable number of patients.

Although there is no statistically significant difference in the analgesic activity between the two drugs there is some evidence that pain relief lasts longer with diflunisal than with glafenine. Undoubtedly, the psychological factor has been very important in this trial as the impact of close follow-up by the doctor in the status of the patient's condition cannot be overlooked.

Both drugs have been safe and the fact that two patients of the glafenine group vomited 10 min after administration of the drug was considered as symptomatic and evaluated as non-clinically significant.

Summary

The analgesic activity of diflunisal (250 mg) versus glafenine (400 mg) as a single oral dose has been studied in cancer patients with moderate to severe pain. Thirty-six patients have so far been entered to the study—19 in the diflunisal group and 17 in the glafenine group. There were three drop-outs, two in the glafenine group who were not evaluated because of vomiting 10 min after the administration of the drug and the third in the diflunisal group who experienced withdrawal symptoms after having been withdrawn from his routine analgesic treatment with dextropropoxyphene.

Both drugs showed significant analgesic activity since only one patient from each group showed no improvement of pain. Eleven out of 18 in the diflunisal group and seven of 15 in the glafenine group were free of pain 10 h after administration of the drug. The remaining six patients of the diflunisal group and seven of the glafenine group experienced relief of pain from 1 to 8 h.

Zusammenfassung

Es wurde die analgesische Wirksamkeit von Diflunisal (250 mg) gegenüber Glanphenin (400 mg) als einzelne orale Dosis in Krebspatienten mit mäßigem bis heftigem Schmerz untersucht. Sechsunddreißig Patienten sind bisher in diese Studie einbezogen worden—19 in der Diflunisal-Gruppe, und 17 in der Glaphenin-Gruppe. Es gab drei Ausfälle: zwei in der Glaphenin-Gruppe, die nicht ausgewertet wurden, weil sie sich zehn Minuten nach der Verabreichung der Droge übergaben, und der Dritte in der Diflunisal-Gruppe, der Entziehungssymptome verspürte, nachdem er von seiner routinemäßigen analgesischen Behandlung mit Dextropropoxyphen weggenommen worden war.

Beide Drogen zeigten eine bedeutsame analgesische Wirksamkeit, da nur ein Patient aus jeder Gruppe keine Verminderung des Schmerzes verzeichnete. Elf von achtzehn in der Diflunisal-Gruppe und sieben von fünfzehn in der Glaphenin-Gruppe waren 10 Stunden nach Verabreichung der Droge schmerzfrei. Die restlichen sechs Patienten der Diflunisal-Gruppe verspürten innerhalb 1 bis 8 Stunden eine Linderung des Schmerzes.

Résumé

On étudie l'activité analgésique comparée du diflunisal (250 mg) et de la glafénine (400 mg) en une seule dose par voie orale sur des malades cancéreux souffrant de douleurs modérées à aiguës. L'étude a porté jusqu'ici sur 36 malades: 19 dans le groupe "diflunisal", 17 dans le groupe "glafénine". Deux des malades du groupe "glafénine" ont été exclus de l'étude parce qu'ils vomissaient dix minutes après administration du médicament, et un des malades du groupe "diflunisal" a été exclu de l'étude parce qu'il présentait des symptômes de manque après suppression de son traitement habituel par le dextropropoxyphène.

Les deux médicaments présentent une activité analgésique significative, car un seul malade de chaque groupe n'est pas soulagé. 11 malades sur 18 du groupe "diflunisal" et 7 malades sur 15 groupe du "glafénine" sont entièrement soulagés pendant dix heures après administration du médicament. Les six malades restants du groupe "diflunisal" et les sept du groupe "glafénine" éprouvent un soulagement d'une durée de 1 à 8 heures.

Sommario

In pazienti affetti da cancro con dolori da lievi a vivi se è studiata l'efficacia analgesica del diflunisal (250 mg) nei confronti della glafenina (400 mg) somministrati in dose orale unica. Finora hanno preso parte allo studio trentasei pazienti: 19 nel gruppo diflunisal e 17 nel gruppo glafenina. Si sono verificati tre ritiri, due nel gruppo glafenina per via di vomito dieci minuti dopo la somministrazione del medicinale e uno nel gruppo diflunisal per sintomi di privazione dopo averlo tolto dal suo trattamento abituale con un altro analgesico, il destropropossifene.

Entrambi i medicamenti hanno mostrato un notevole effetto analgesico dato che solo un paziente di ciascun gruppo non mostrò alcuna attenuazione del dolore. Nel gruppo diflunisal 11 pazienti su 18 e nel gruppo glafenina 7 pazienti su 15 non sentirono più alcun dolore per dieci ore dopo la somministrazione dei medicamenti. I restanti sei pazienti del gruppo diflunisal e sette del gruppo glafenina mostrarono una riduzione del dolore per il periode de 1 a 8 ore.

Resumen

Se ha estudiado la actividad analgésica del diflunisal (250 mg) y la glafenina (400 mg) en dosis oral única en pacientes cancerosos con dolor moderado on intenso. Hasta ahora han participado en el estudio 36 pacientes; 19 en el grupo del diflunisal y 17 en el de la glafenina. Se retiraron tres pacientes del estudio, dos en el grupo de glafenina debido a vómito a los 10 minutos de la administración del medicamento y el tercero en el grupo del diflunisal, debido a síntomas de abstinencia luego de la interrupción de su tratamiento analgésico rutinario con dextropropoxifeno.

Ambos medicamentos tuvieron una actividad analgésica importante, ya que sólo un paciente en cada grupo no experimentó mejoría del dolor. Once de los 18 en el grupo del diflunisal y 7 de los 15 en el de la glafenina no tuvieron dolor durante 10 horas, luego de la administración de los medicamentos. Los restantes pacientes, 6 en el grupo del diflunisal y 7 en el de la glafenina tuvieron alivio del dolor por periodos de 1 a 8 horas.

Sumário

A actividade analgésica do diflunisal (250 mg) comparado com a glafenina (400 mg), numa única dose oral, foi estudada em doentes cancerosos com dor moderada a severa. Trinta e seis doentes foram, até agora, incluídos neste estudo—19 no grupo diflunisal e 17 no grupo glafenina. Houve três casos eliminados—dois deles no grupo glafenina que não foram avaliados devido a terem vomitado dez minutos depois da administração do medicamento, e o terceiro no grupo diflunisal devido a este doente ter desenvolvido sintomas reactivos de suspensão depois de ter parado de tomar o analgésico que tomava como rotina—neste caso o dextropropoxifeno.

Ambas as drogas mostraram ter uma significativa actividade analgésica, visto que apenas um doente de cada grupo não sentiu qualquer alívio da dor. Onze de 18 doentes no grupo diflunisal e sete de 15 doentes no grupo glafenina ficaram absolutamente sem dor 10 horas depois da administração da droga. Os restantes seis doentes do grupo diflunisal e sete do grupo glafenina sentiram alívio da dor durante 1 a 8 horas.

Diflunisal compared with Pentazocine in Cancer Pain

M. HAYAT and M. DELGADO

*Institut Gustave Roussy,
Villejuif, France*

Control of cancer pain is a major problem and during the evolution of the disease various analgesics are frequently prescribed. There is, however, a need for a new drug with long-acting efficacy and with few or no side-effects but in cancerology any new analgesic should be at least as active as one of the well-known potent analgesics. This study compares the efficacy of diflunisal with that of pentazocine.

Material and Methods

The study was controlled, single-blind, randomized and single dose, comparing the efficacy of 500 mg diflunisal with 50 mg pentazocine. Forty in-patients with moderate to severe cancer pain (pulmonary carcinoma, lymphoma or bone metastases) entered the study and those who were excluded had hypersensitivity to salicylates or were currently taking oral anti-coagulants or hypoglycaemics. Those with peptic ulcer or gastrointestinal haemorrhage within the last two years were also excluded.

No other analgesic was to be administered within the 4 h prior to the administration of the test medication and no other analgesic or anti-inflammatory agent could be given during the study. When the use of another analgesic became inevitable, the case was considered as a failure.

Prior to taking the test medication the patient recorded the intensity of spontaneous pain. Evaluation was made after 1, 2, 4, 6, 8 and if possible 10 h. The patient assessment was collected by the same investigator throughout the study.

The evaluation was made according to two modalities:
   (1) spontaneous pain: graded as none, mild, moderate or severe;
   (2) pain relief: by a visual analogue scale. Score was recorded on a continuous line marked "no relief" at one end and "complete relief" at the other.

Pre-treatment characteristics of the patients are shown in Table 1. The score of pre-treatment spontaneous pain showed that of 20 patients taking diflunisal, 18 had severe and two moderate pain compared to 16 and four respectively in the pentazocine group.

Diflunisal: Royal Society of Medicine International Congress and Symposium Series No. 6, published jointly by Academic Press Inc. (London) Ltd., and the Royal Society of Medicine.

Table 1

Pre-treatment characteristics age and sex

	< 30	Age (years) 30–59	> 60	Total
Diflunisal				
Male	5	7	0	12
Female	2	3	3	8
Pentazocine				
Male	—	6	1	7
Female	1	9	3	13

No statistically significant differences.

Results

Forty patients were randomly allocated to the diflunisal group or pentazocine group. Categories of change in the two groups were defined as follows:
- no pain: disappearance of pain;
- improved: pain still present but rated less severe than at pre-treatment;
- no improvement: no change to pain rating, pain rate more severe than at pre-treatment or patient dropped out due to ineffective therapy.

Two patients in the diflunisal group and five in the pentazocine group discontinued the study after 4 h due to a lack of therapeutic response. At 2 h, 50% of the patients in the diflunisal group and 45% in the pentazocine group had no pain. At 8 h, 80% of the patients in diflunisal group and 70% in pentazocine had no pain. There is no statistically significant difference between the two treatment groups. Patients who discontinued due to lack of therapeutic response were not considered in this analysis. The treatment groups do not differ significantly in the pain relief.

Two patients on pentazocine and one on diflunisal had adverse reactions, but none was serious (Table 2).

Table 2

Side-effects

Treatment group	Adverse clinical effect(s)	Number of patient	Duration
Diflunisal	Shivering and increased arterial pressure	1	2 h
Pentazocine	Vomiting	1	1 h
	Nausea	1	2 h

Discussion and Conclusion

The result of this study made on 40 patients indicates that a single dose of diflunisal 500 mg is as active as a single dose of pentazocine 50 mg.

A statistical analysis was not possible but we did not observe a difference in this trial made on 40 patients. It is possible that, with a different dosage, or with more patients, a difference may appear, but a higher dosage may induce more adverse effects, and if more patients are needed to observe a difference, it means that this difference is small.

In conclusion, this study demonstrates that the relief of cancer pain by diflunisal and pentazocine is similar.

Summary

The analgesic efficacy and the safety of single doses of 500 mg of diflunisal and 50 mg of pentazocine were compared in a single-blind pilot study in patients suffering from pain due to malignant disease. Forty patients with moderate to severe pain due to pulmonary carcinoma, lymphoma or bone metastases were randomly allocated to the treatment groups (20 in each group).

The treatment groups were comparable with regard to all pre-treatment characteristics. Efficacy was evaluated by analysing spontaneous pain and pain relief by the visual analogue scale recorded before treatment and at 1, 2, 4, 6, 8 and 10 h. Efficacy was good and comparable for both drugs and no statistically significant differences were found. However, two patients on diflunisal and five on pentazocine were given alternative pain medication due to a lack of response and were considered as failures. Tolerance was excellent in both groups except one on diflunisal and two on pentazocine who reported slight adverse reaction.

Zusammenfassung

Es wurden die analgesische Wirksamkeit und die Sicherheit von Einzeldosen von 500 mg Diflunisal und 50 mg Pentazocine in einer einfach blinden Studie in Patienten verglichen, die an Schmerzen infolge von Krebs litten. Vierzig Patienten mit mäßigem bis heftigem Schmerz infolge von Lungenkrebs, Lymphom oder Knochenmetastase wurden den Behandlungsgruppen wahllos zugeteilt (20 in jeder Gruppe).

Die Behandlungsgruppen waren in bezug auf alle Vorbehandlungscharakteristiken vergleichbar. Die Wirksamkeit wurde durch Analysieren von Spontanschmerz und Schmerzlinderung durch die optische Analogskala ausgewertet, die vor der Behandlung und bei 1, 2, 4, 6, 8 and 10 Stunden aufgezeichnet wurde. Die Wirksamkeit war gut und für beide Drogen vergleichbar, und es wurden keine bedeutsamen Unterschiede festgestellt. 2 Patienten auf Diflunisal und 5 auf Pentazocin erhielten jedoch wegen mangelnder Reation alternative Schmerzlinderungsmittel und wurden als Versager vermerkt. Die Verträglichkeit war in beiden Gruppen ausgezeichnet, ausgenommen einer auf Diflunisal und zwei auf Pentazocine, die eine geringfügige widrige Reaktion meldeten.

Résumé

On compare l'efficacité analgésique et l'innocuité de doses uniques de 500 mg de diflunisal et 50 mg de pentazocine dans une étude pilote à simple anonymat sur des malades souffrant de douleurs dues à une tumeur cancéreuse. On répartit au hasard en deux groupes de vingt quarante malades souffrant de douleurs modérées à aiguës dues à un cancer du poumon, à un lymphome ou à des métastases osseuses.

Les deux groupes sont comparables par toutes leurs caractéristiques antérieures au traitement. On évalue l'efficacité en analysant la douleur spontanée et le soulagement de la douleur par l'échelle visuelle analogique enregistrée avant traitement et 1, 2, 4, 6, 8 et 10 heures après traitement. L'efficacité est bonne et comparable pour les deux médicaments, et on ne constate aucune différence statistiquement significative. Toutefois, deux malades du groupe "diflunisal" et cinq malades du groupe "pentazocine" ont reçu d'autres analgésiques faute de réaction, et leurs cas ont été considérés comme des échecs. La tolérance est excellente dans les deux groupes, sauf pour un malade du groupe "diflunisal" et deux malades du groupe "pentazocine" qui présentaient de légères réactions défavorables.

Sommario

In uno studio pilota "single-blind" su pazienti affetti da dolori da tumori maligni si mise a raffronto l'efficacia analgesica e la sicurezza del diflunisal in dose unica da 500 mg con quella della pentazocina in dose unica da 50 mg. Quaranta pazienti affetti da dolori da lievi ad intensi a causa di carcinoma polmonare, limfoma oppure metastasi ossee furono ripartiti a caso nei due gruppi di trattamento (20 ciascun gruppo).

I due gruppi erano simili per quanto riguarda tutte le caratteristiche di pretrattamento. L'efficacia venne valutata analizzando il dolore spontaneo e il sollievo dal dolore a mezzo della scala visiva analogica registrata prima del trattamento ed alle ore 1, 2, 4, 6, 8 e 10. L'efficacia fu buona e simile per entrambi i medicamenti e non si trovò alcuna differenza statisticamente significativa. Tuttavia, per mancanza di effetto analgesico, a due pazienti del gruppo diflunisal e a 5 del gruppo pentazocina furono somministrati altri farmaci. Questi casi vennero considerati insuccessi. La tolleranza fu ottima in entrambi i gruppi eccetto per un paziente del diflunisal e due della pentazocina i quali denunciarono leggere reazioni avverse.

Resumen

Se comparó la eficacia analgésica de una dosis única de 500 mg de diflunisal y 50 mg de pentazocina en un estudio piloto ciego en pacientes con dolor debido a una enfermedad maligna. Se distribuyeron al azar 40 pacientes (en dos grupos de 20) con dolor moderado o intenso debido a carcinoma de pulmón, linfoma o metástasis ósea.

Los pacientes eran todos comparables en cuanto a sus características previas al tratamiento. Se evaluó la eficacia analizando el dolor espontáneo y el alivio del dolor por medio de una escala visual analógica utilizada antes del tratamiento y a la primera, segunda, cuarta, sexta, octava y décima horas después del mismo. El grado de eficacia fue satisfactorio y comparable para ambos medicamentos y no se encontraron diferencias notables. Sin embargo, 2 pacientes con diflunisal y 5 con pentazocina tuvieron que recibir otros analgésicos debido a la falta de reacción y se consideraron, por lo tanto, fracasos terapéuticos. Hubo excelente tolerancia para ambos grupos, excepto un paciente con diflunisal y 2 con pentazocina que señalaron una reacción adversa leve.

Sumário

A eficácia analgésica e grau de segurança de doses únicas de 500 mg de diflunisal e 50 mg de pentazocina foram comparadas num estudo-piloto às cegas, efectuado em doentes sofrendo de dor devida a doença maligna. Quarenta doentes com dor moderada a severa devida a carcinoma pulmonar, linfoma ou metástases ósseas, foram repartidos ao acaso entre os grupos de tratamento (20 doentes em cada grupo).

Os grupos de tratamento eram comparáveis em relação a todas as características pré-tratamento. A eficácia foi avaliada por análise de dor espontânea e alívio da dor mediante uma escala analógica visual, e os registos foram efectuados antes do tratamento e 1, 2, 4, 6, 8 e 10 horas após tratamento. A eficácia foi boa e comparável para ambas as drogas, não se tendo verificado quaisquer diferenças de significado estatístico. Contudo, 2 doentes do grupo diflunisal e 5 do grupo pentazocina tiveram de tomar analgésicos alternativos por não terem reagido às drogas em estudo, e foram considerados como fracassos. A tolerância foi excelente em ambos os grupos, com excepção de 1 doente no grupo diflunisal e 2 no grupo pentazocina que se queixaram de ligeiras reacções adversas.

Diflunisal in the Treatment of Cancer Pain

ITALIAN COMMITTEE FOR THE STUDY AND TREATMENT OF CANCER PAIN *

The Italian Committee for the Study and Treatment of Cancer Pain has supervised a trial comparing the analgesic affects of a single oral dose of diflunisal (500 mg) versus aspirin (800 mg). This randomized study was conducted in a double-blind crossover manner with clinical assessment performed hourly for 8 h using a rating scale and the Huskisson visual analogue scale.

One hundred and fourteen patients of both sexes (age range 18–70 years) who had advanced solid tumours entered the study and were allocated to one of two treatment groups matched for age, sex and clinical history. No patient had had specific analgesic or general therapy in the two weeks prior to the start of the trial and the life expectancy in all cases was greater than two months.

The overall incidence of adverse reactions was higher in the aspirin group and considering only gastro-intestinal side effects, this difference was statistically significant ($P<0.01$) in favour of diflunisal. Pain relief, evaluated on the Huskisson visual analogue scale was greater in the diflunisal group, the differences being highly significant in the period between 6 and 8 h post-dosing. Various analyses applied to the crossover design showed,

(1) there were no statistically significant differences between the two groups in terms of age, sex, etc;

(2) patients showed a similar drug response regardless of administration sequence;

(3) diflunisal was significantly more effective as evaluated by analogue and semantic scales;

(4) side-effects, particularly gastric disturbances, were significantly lower in the diflunisal group and this is a very important factor in treating this type of patient in whom gastric tolerance is generally very poor.

The Italian Clinical Committee for the study and treatment of cancer pain believes strongly that diflunisal is a useful drug in this type of patient and further studies are in progress to evaluate the role of this drug in long-term therapy.

---

*Institute Nazionale Tumori, Milano; Ospedale Malpighi, Bologna; Centre Oncologico, Ancona; Institute Chimica Farmaceutica, Roma; Ospedale Civile, Gubbie; Institute Regina Elena, Roma. (Paper presented by Professor V. Ventafridda.)

Diflunisal: Royal Society of Medicine International Congress and Symposium Series No. 6, published jointly by Academic Press Inc. (London) Ltd., and the Royal Society of Medicine.

Summary

One hundred and fourteen cancer patients received either diflunisal (500 mg) or aspirin (800 mg) in a single daily oral dose for the treatment of pain. The double-blind study was organized on a multi-centred basis and all patients treated had advanced solid tumours. Diflunisal was significantly more effective than aspirin and side effects, particularly gastric disturbances, were also less frequent when diflunisal was taken. Further studies into the use of this drug in cancer patients are in progress.

Zusammenfassung

Einhundertvierzehn Krebspatienten erhielten entweder Diflunisal (500 mg) oder Aspirin (800 mg) in einer einzigen täglichen oralen Dosis zur Behandlung des Schmerzes. Die doppelt blinde Studie wurde auf einer mehrzentrigen Grundlage organisiert, und alle behandelten Patienten hatten fortgeschrittene feste Tumore. Diflunisal war bedeutend wirksamer als Aspirin, und Nebenwirkungen—besonders gastrische Störungen—waren ebenfalls weniger häufig, wenn Diflunisal eingenommen wurde. Weitere Untersuchungen der Verwendung dieser Droge in Krebskranken befinden sich in der Durchführung.

Résumé

Cent quatorze malades cancéreux reçoivent soit 500 mg de diflunisal, soit 800 mg d'aspirine en une seule dose orale journalière pour le traitement de la douleur. L'étude à double anonymat est organisée de manière pluricentrique, et tous les malades ont des tumeurs compactes avancées. Le diflunisal est significativement plus efficace que l'aspirine et ses effets secondaires, en particulier les désordres gastriques, sont moins fréquents. De nouvelles études sur l'emploi de ce médicament sur les cancéreux sont en cours.

Sommario

A 114 pazienti affetti da cancro si somministrò come analgesico o 500 mg di diflunisal o 800 mg di aspirina in unica dose giornaliera. Lo studio è stato del tipo "double-blind" pluricentrato e tutti i pazienti trattati presentavano tumori solidi in stato avanzato. Il diflunisal si rivelò notevolmente più efficace dell'aspirina e gli effetti secondari, particolarmente i disturbi gastrici, furono meno frequenti con il diflunisal. Sono in corso ulteriori studi sull'uso di questo medicamento su pazienti affetti da cancro.

Resumen

Se administró diflunisal (500 mg) o aspirina (800 mg) en una sola dosis oral diaria para aliviar el dolor a ciento catorce pacientes con cáncer. Este estudio se realizó a doble ciego en múltiples centros y todos los pacientes en tratamiento tenían tumores avanzados importantes. El diflunisal demostró ser bastante más eficaz que la aspirina y los efectos secundarios, especialmente las perturbaciones gástricas, fueron menos frecuentes con diflunisal. Actualmente se prosiguen los estudios acerca del uso de este medicamento en los pacientes con cáncer.

Sumário

Cento e catorze doentes cancerosos receberam quer diflunisal (500 mg) quer aspirina (800 mg) numa única dose diá.ia o al, para alívio de dor. O estudo, duplamente às cegas, foi organizado numa base de multi-centros, e todos os doentes tratados tinham tumores sólidos em estado avançado. O diflunisal foi significativamente mais eficaz do que a aspirina, e os efeitos secundários, particularmente perturbações gástricas, foram menos frequentes quando os doentes tomaram diflunisal. Novos estudos sobre o uso desta droga em doentes cancerosos estão presentemente em curso.

Effect of Twice Daily Diflunisal on Gastrointestinal Blood Loss

P. J. DE SCHEPPER and T. B. TJANDRAMAGA

Department of Pharmacology, University of Leuven,
Leuven, Belgium

Gastric erosions and occult blood loss exceeding the physiological amount of 0·5–1·5 ml per day in man has been well documented following the administration of acetylsalicylic acid (ASA) and most other nonsteroidal anti-inflammatory/analgesic drugs. This effect, which seems to be dose-dependent, has, in the case of ASA, been shown to be enhanced by the concomitant ingestion of rather substantial amounts of ethanol. Diflunisal, a non-acetylated salicylic acid derivative with rather potent analgesic/anti-inflammatory properties did not produce superficial haemorrhagic areas in the rat gastric mucosa when given in doses up to 25 times larger than those needed to inhibit carrageenan induced foot oedema. It therefore seemed to be worthwhile examining the effect of clinically relevant doses of this new drug upon occult faecal blood loss in man.

In two previous controlled double-blind studies (De Schepper, 1978) in normal volunteers, it had been shown that diflunisal 250 mg b.i.d. did not significantly increase occult blood loss versus control while ASA at 600 or 750 mg q.i.d. had a significant effect (Table 1). In addition, it was shown that there was no significant enhancement of faecal blood loss when ethanol was administered in combination with diflunisal during two consecutive days. The effect of ASA on faecal blood loss, however, was significantly enhanced by the addition of ethanol. In view of these

Table 1

Mean faecal blood loss during ASA or diflunisal treatment

Treatment	Dose	Group I[a] Control	Group I[a] Treatment	Group II[a] Control	Group II[a] Treatment
Diflunisal	250 mg b.i.d.	0·26 ml	0·32 ml	0·42 ml	0·53 ml
ASA	600–750 mg q.i.d.	0·39 ml	6·87 ml	0·86 ml	3·20 ml

[a] Crossover design.

Diflunisal: Royal Society of Medicine International Congress and Symposium Series No. 6, published jointly by Academic Press Inc. (London) Ltd., and the Royal Society of Medicine.

results and since doses up to 500 mg b.i.d. of diflunisal have since been recommended, a third study was performed with the objective to compare faecal blood loss during the administration of diflunisal 500 mg b.i.d. and of placebo.

Methods

A single-blind two-period crossover study without washout was performed in 12 normal male volunteers who had no obvious or previous history of gastrointestinal bleeding or lesions. The subjects were randomly assigned to two groups of six. Three days before the start of the study 100μCi of ^{51}Cr labelled autologous red cells were administered to each subject. The study consisted of four periods:

Day 1–5
No-drug pre-treatment control period.

Day 6–12
Six subjects received diflunisal 500 mg at 8 a.m. and 8 p.m. and six received placebo.

Day 13–19
Subjects switched to the alternative treatment.

Day 20–26
Post-treatment follow-up period, all subjects received placebo.

The average daily faecal blood loss was computed using samples from days 1 to 5, 8 to 12, 15 to 19, 20 to 22, 25 and 26. Blood samples were taken at regular intervals throughout the study to establish the decay curve of plasma radioactivity and to monitor plasma levels of diflunisal.

Results

The mean daily faecal blood loss of all subjects during the pre-treatment control period was 0·80 ml (Table 2). During diflunisal treatment the mean daily faecal blood

Table 2

Mean daily faecal blood loss

Trial period	Faecal blood loss (ml)
Control	0·81
Placebo	1·00
Diflunisal	0·93
Follow-up (1)	0·73
Follow-up (2)	1·12

loss was 0·93 ml, while during placebo treatment it was 1·00 ml. These values were statistically indistinguishable. Similarly, there was no statistically significant difference between the mean daily faecal blood loss during the pre-treatment control period and during the post-treatment periods. Non-parametric procedures were used in the statistical analysis of the data. All statistical tests were performed at the 5% level of significance.

Diflunisal plasma levels indicated that all subjects adhered to the prescribed treatment and no adverse effects on laboratory data and no adverse clinical effects were noted.

Discussion

When bleeding was seen in patients taking diflunisal it was extremely irregular, some showing 30–35 ml one day and none the next. This is not at all like the bleeding seen with ASA which is different both in quantity and quality, taking up to 10 days after withdrawal of ASA before the bleeding stops.

Previous studies have shown that diflunisal 250 mg b.i.d. did not induce gastrointestinal microbleeding as observed with ASA. From the present study it may be concluded that diflunisal 500 mg b.i.d. does not increase faecal blood loss above control values in normal volunteers.

Reference

De Schepper, P. J. (1978). *Clin. Pharmac. Ther.* (In press).

Summary

Three faecal blood loss studies were performed in normal volunteers using ^{51}Cr labelled red cells. In two previous double-blind studies where diflunisal (250 mg b.i.d.) was compared with acetylsalicylic acid (ASA) with and without ethanol, diflunisal did not significantly alter physiological blood loss but this was significantly increased following ASA. The effect was further enhanced by the addition of ethanol.

In view of the current clinical use of diflunisal in a 500 mg b.i.d. dose, a third study was performed comparing this higher dose level with placebo. This was a single-blind crossover study in 12 normal subjects. After a 5-day pre-treatment control period during which physiological blood loss was measured, six subjects received diflunisal and six placebo during 7 days. Subjects were then switched to the alternative treatment during 7 days, and this was followed by a 7-day placebo treatment in all subjects. Mean faecal blood loss in all subjects during the control period was 0·80 ml/day; blood loss values during placebo and diflunisal treatment were 1·00 ml/day and 0·93 ml/day, respectively. Statistical treatment showed that faecal blood loss values during all periods were indistinguishable.

It is concluded that diflunisal up to 500 mg b.i.d. has no significant effect upon gastrointestinal blood loss in normal volunteers.

Zusammenfassung

Es wurden drei Kotblutverlustudien in normalen Freiwilligen unter Benutzung von mit ^{51}CR gekennzeichneten roten Zellen durchgeführt. In zwei vorangegangenen doppelt blinden Studien wurde Diflunisal (250 mg zweimal täglich) mit Azetylsalizylsäure (ASA) mit und ohne Äthanol verglichen; Diflunisal erbrachte keine bedeutsame Änderung des physiologischen Blutverlustes, jedoch wurde dieser im Anschluß an ASA bedeutend erhöht. Der Effekt wurde durch die Hinzugabe von Äthanol noch weiter verstärkt.

In Anbetracht der derzeitigen klinischen Benutzung von Diflunisal in einer Dosis von 500 mg zweimal täglich wurde eine höhere dritte Studie durchgeführt, in der dieser Dosenstand mit Placebo verglichen wurde. Hierbei handelte es sich um eine einfach blinde Austauschstudie in zwölf normalen Personen. Nach einer fünftägigen Vorbehandlungs-Kontrollzeit, während der der physiologische Blutverlust gemessen wurde, erhielten sechs Personen sieben Tage lang Diflunisal, und sechs Placebo, und daian Diflunisal und sechs Placebo und daran schloß sich eine siebentägige Placebo-Behandlung in allen Personen an. Der mittlere Kotblutverlust in allen Personen während des Kontrollzeitraumes betrug 0,80 ml/Tag; die Blutverlustwerte während der Placebo- und Diflunisal-Behandlung betrugen 1,00 ml/Tage bzw. 0,93 ml/Tage. Die statistische Behandlung zeigte, daß die Kotblutverlustwerte während aller Zeiträume nicht zu unterscheiden waren.

Es wird gefolgert, daß Diflunisal bis zu 500 mg zweimal täglich keine bedeutsame Auswirkung auf den gastrointestinalen Blutverlust in normalen Freiwilligen hat.

Résumé

On fait trois études sur la présence de sang dans les excréments chez des volontaires normaux, à l'aide de globules rouges marqués au ^{51}Cr. Dans deux études précédentes à double anonymat, oú l'on a comparé le diflunisal (2×250 mg par jour) et l'acide acétylsalicylique avec ou sans éthanol, on a constaté que le diflunisal ne modiffe pas significativement la perte de sang physiologique, laquelle augmente au contraire significativement avec l'acide acétylsalicylique. L'effet est encore accru par addition d'éthanol.

Compte tenu de l'emploi clinique actuel du diflunisal à raison de 2×500 mg par jour, on fait une troisème étude pour comparer les effets de cette posologie supérieure à ceux d'un placebo. Il s'agit d'une étude croisée à simple anonymat sur douze sujets normaux. Après une période de pré-traitement de cinq jours pendant laquelle on mesure la perte de sang physiologique, six sujets reçoivent du diflunisal et six du placebo pendant sept jours. Les sujets sont ensuite soumis au traitement d'étude pendant sept jours, puis à un traitement par placebo pendant sept jours. La perte de sang dans les excréments est de 0,80 ml/j pour tous les sujets pendant la période préliminaire, 1,00 ml/j pendant le traitement au placebo et 0,93 ml/j pendant le traitement au diflunisal. Le traitement statistique des résultats montre que les valeurs des pertes de sang dans les excréments pendant toutes les périodes sont indiscernables.

On en conclut que l'administration de 2×500 mg par jour de diflunisal n'a aucun effet significatif sur les pertes de sang gastro-intestinales chez des volontaires normaux.

Sommario

In volontari normali si effettuarono tre studi sulla perdita di sangue fecale impiegando globuli rossi all'isotopo ^{51}CR. In due precedenti studi "double-blind" in cui si mise a raffronto il diflunisal (250 mg due volte al giorno) con l'acido acetilsalicilico (AAS) con e senza etanolo, il diflunisal non cambiò in modo significativo la perdita di sangue fisiologica, mentre questa aumentò notevolmente con l'acido acetilsalicilico. Tale effetto si intensificò con l'aggiunta dell'etanolo.

In vista del corrente uso clinico del diflunisal in dosi da 500 mg due volte al giorno, si eseguì un terzo studio comparando tale più elevata dose con un placebo. Si trattò di uno studio "single-blind" con scambio in 12 soggetti normali. Dopo un periodo di controllo pretrattamento di cinque giorni durante il quale si misurò la perdita di sangue fisiologica, 6 soggetti ricevettero il diflunisal e 6 il placebo, per sette giorni. I soggetti vennero quindi passati al trattamento alternativo durante sette giorni, a cui si fece seguire, per tutti i soggetti, un trattamento di sette giorni con placebo. In tutti i soggetti la perdita di sangue media durante il periodo di controllo fu di 0,80 ml/giorno; i valori durante il trattamento con placebo e diflunisal furono rispettivamente di 1,00 e 0,93 ml/giorno. Il trattamento statistico mostrò che non vi era alcuna differenza distinguibile tra i valori di perdita di sangue fecale durante tutti i periodi.

Si conclude che, in dosi fino a 500 mg due volte al giorno, il diflunisal non ha alcun effetto significativo sulla perdita di sangue gastro-intestinale in soggetti normali.

Resumen

Se realizaron tres estudios con voluntarios en buen estado de salud para investigar pérdidas de sangre en la materia fecal usando glóbulos rojos marcados con Cr 51. En dos estudios a doble ciego realizados previamente en los que el diflunisal (250 mg tres veces por día) se comparó con el ácido acetilsalicílico (AAS) con y sin etanol, el diflunisal no produjo ninguna alteración notable en la pérdida fisiológica de sangre, mientras que hubo considerable aumento en la pérdida sanguínea con la administración del ácido acetilsalicílico. Este efecto se acentuó al añadir etanol. Teniendo en cuenta el actual uso clínico del diflunisal en dosis de 500 mg dos veces por día se realizó un tercer estudio comparando el diflunisal en esta dosis con un placebo. Este fue un estudio cruzado a ciego con doce personas normales. Se dio diflunisal a 6 personas y placebo a las otras 6 durante 7 días, luego de un periodo de control de de 5 días antes del tratamiento, en el cual se midió la pérdida fisiológica de sangre. A continuación, se cambió el tratamiento de todos los participantes al otro medicamento y finalmente se terminó con un periodo de 7 días de tratamiento con placebo para todos los voluntarios. El promedio de la pérdida de sangre en la materia fecal de todos los participantes durante el periodo de control fue de 0,80 ml/día y las pérdidas durante el tratamiento con placebo y diflunisal fueron de 1,00 ml/día y 0,93 ml/día, respectivamente. El análisis estadístico de los datos obtenidos demostró que los valores de pérdida sanguínea fecal durante todos los periodos no presentaban diferencias. La conclusión es que el diflunisal en dosis máximas de 500 mg dos veces al día apenas influye sobre la pérdida gastrointestinal de sangre en voluntarios de salud normal.

Sumário

Três estudos sobre perdas sanguíneas fecais foram efectuados em voluntários normais, usando glóbulos vermelhos marcados com ^{51}Cr. Em dois estudos precedentes, duplamente às cegas, em que o diflunisal (250 mg 2 vezes/dia) foi comparado com o ácido acetilsalicílico (ASA) com e sem etanol, o diflunisal não alterou significativamente a perda sanguínea fisiológica, mas esta perda aumentou significativamente após ingestão de ASA. Este efeito era ainda mais acentuado pela adição de etanol.

Em vista do corrente uso clínico de diflunisal numa dose de 500 mg 2 vezes/dia, foi efectuado um terceiro estudo comparando este nível mais alto de dose com um placebo. Este estudo foi efectuado segundo um sistema cruzado, às cegas, em doze indivíduos normais. Após um período de contrôle de cinco dias antes do tratamento, durante o qual foi medida a perda sanguínea fisiológica, seis indivíduos receberam diflunisal e os outros seis um placebo, durante sete dias. Os indivíduos foram então trocados e postos no tratamento alternativo durante sete dias, seguindo-se mais sete dias em que todos os indivíduos receberam o placebo. A média da perda sanguínea fecal em todos os indivíduos durante o período de contrôle era, 0,80 ml/dia; os valores da perda sanguínea durante o tratamento com placebo e com diflunisal foram 1,00 ml/dia e 0,93 ml/dia, respectivamente. A análise estatística revelou que os valores de perda sanguínea fecal durante todos os períodos eram indeferenciáveis.

Concluiu-se pois que o diflunisal, em doses até 500 mg duas vezes por dia, não produz qualquer efeito significativo sobre a perda sanguínea gastro-intestinal em voluntários normais.

Diflunisal in General Practice

E. C. HUSKISSON

St Bartholomew's Hospital, London, England

Trial Design

Five hundred general practitioners cooperated in studying five patients each, treated either with aspirin or diflunisal for five days. The method has been described in detail elsewhere (Huskisson, 1978). Aspirin was given in a dose of 600 mg q.i.d., diflunisal in an initial dose of 500 mg, then either 250 or 500 mg daily according to response. An attempt was made to conceal the identity of the treatment from both doctor and patient. Patients studied had a variety of conditions of which sprains, strains and osteoarthritis were the commonest.

Results

A total of 967 patients received diflunisal and 935 received aspirin. Global assessment of response by both doctor and patient showed diflunisal to be superior to aspirin. Side-effects were not particularly common in either group but gastric side-effects significantly commoner and more severe with aspirin than with diflunisal. Patients were more often withdrawn from aspirin therapy during the study. The dose of aspirin was kept constant in most patients; that of diflunisal was equally often 250 and 500 mg twice daily. The dose of diflunisal did not influence either effectiveness or side-effects.

Conclusions

Diflunisal is an effective analgesic and for use in general practice, doses of 250 or 500 mg b.i.d. are required. In this study it had four advantages over aspirin. It was more effective, less toxic, less often withdrawn and given only twice daily. It will be useful in general practice for conditions which require either a short course of drug therapy or chronic administration.

Reference

Hiskisson, E. C. (1978).

Summary

Diflunisal was compared with acetylsalicylic acid (ASA) as a simple analgesic in almost 2000 patients in general practice. The patients had a variety of painful syndromes for which a simple analgesic would have been prescribed. They were given either diflunisal 500 mg stat, then 250 or 500 mg b.i.d. or ASA 600 mg q.i.d. The ASA was pink and called "DQ 174" in order to obscure its nature. Treatment was continued for 5 days.

Diflunisal was superior to ASA, caused fewer gastric side effects and was less often withdrawn during the study. It also had the advantage of twice-daily administration. The dosage was as often 250 and 500 mg b.i.d. Diflunisal, therefore, has obvious advantages over ASA as an analgesic in general practice.

Zusammenfassung

Diflunisal wurde in nahezu 2000 Patienten in Allgemeinpraxis als einfaches Analgetikum mit Azetylsalizylsäure (ASA) verglichen. Die Patienten hatten eine Vielzahl schmerzhafter Syndrome, für die ein einfaches Analgetikum verschrieben worden wäre. Ihnen wurden entweder Diflunisal 500 mg stat., dann 250 oder 500 mg zweimal täglich, oder ASA 600 mg viermal täglich verabreicht. Die ASA war rosa und trug die Bezeichnung "DQ 174", um ihre Beschaffenheit zu verbergen. Die Behandlung wurde fünf Tage lang fortgesetzt.

Diflunisal war ASA überlegen, verursachte weniger gastrische Nebenwirkungen und wurde während der Studie weniger häufig zurückgezogen. Außerdem hatte es den Vorteil einer zweimal täglichen Verabreichung. Die Dosierung war genau so häufig 250 und 500 mg zweimal täglich. Diflunisal hat daher eindeutige Vorteile gegenüber ASA als Analgetikum in der Allgemeinpraxis.

Résumé

On compare le diflunisal et l'acide acétylsalicylique comme analgésiques simples sur près de 2000 clients de généralistes. Les malades souffrent de syndromes douloureux divers pour lesquels on prescrit un analgésique simple. On leur administre soit 500 mg de diflunisal, puis 2×250 mg ou 2×500 mg de diflunisal par jour, soit 4×600 mg d'acide acétylsalicylique par jour. L'acide acétylsalicylique est rose et est appelé "DQ 174" pour cacher son identité. Le traitement est poursuivi pendant cinq jours.

Le diflunisal est supérieur à l'acide acétylsalicylique, produit moins d'effets secondaires gastriques et est moins souvent retiré pendant l'étude. Il a aussi l'avantage d'être administré deux fois par jour seulement. La dosage atteint souvent 250 ou 500 mg du fois par jour. Le diflunisal a donc des avantages évidents sur l'acide acétylsalicylique en médecine générale.

Sommario

Si è comparato il diflunisal con l'acido acetilsalicilico (AAS) somministrandolo come semplice analgesico in quasi 2.000 pazienti in un ambulatorio di medicina generale. I pazienti rappresentavano varie sindromi dolorose per le quali si sarebbe prescritto un analgesico semplice. A questi fu somministrato o il diflunisal in dose immediata da 500 mg e quindi 250 oppure 500 mg due volte al giorno o dell'AAS in dosi da 600 mg quattro volte al giorno. L'AAS era colorato in rosa e chiamato "DQ 174" al fine di nascondere la sua identità. Il trattamento si estese per cinque giorni.

Il diflunisal si rivelò superiore all'AAS, provocò minori effetti secondari gastrici e subì un numero di ritiri inferiore. Il diflunisal presentava pure il vantaggio della somministrazione due volte al giorno con dosi da 250 oppure 500 mg. Si conclude quindi che il diflunisal presenta ovvi vantaggi nei confronti dell'AAS come analgesico per uso in nella medicina generale.

Resumen

Se comparó el diflunisal con el ácido acetilsalicílico (AAS) como simple analgésico en medicina general con una muestra en 2000 pacientes. Los pacientes presentaban síntomas diversos para los cuales se había recetado un simple analgésico. Se les administró ya sea diflunisal 500 mg al comienzo y luego 250 mg o 500 mg una vez por día o 600 mg de AAS cuatro veces al día. Para ocultar la identidad del AAS se coloreó de rosa y se lo llamó "DQ 174." El tratamiento duró 5 días.

El diflunisal mostró ser superior al AAS, causando menos efectos gástricos secundarios y tuvo que interrumpirse menos veces durante el estudio. También tenía la ventaja de administración dos veces al día. Se usó con la misma frecuencia la dosis de 250 mg como la de 500 mg dos veces por día. Por lo tanto, el diflunisal tiene obvias ventajas sobre el AAS como analgésico para uso en medicina general.

Sumário

O diflunisal foi comparado com o ácido acetilsalicílico (ASA) como um analgésico simples em quase 2000 doentes de clínica geral. Os doentes tinham uma variedade de sindromas dolorosos, para os quais um simples analgésico teria sido receitado. Foi-lhes dado quer diflunisal (500 mg inicial e depois 250 ou 500 mg duas vezes por dia) quer ASA (600 mg quatro vezes por dia). O "ASA" era côr-de-rosa e chamado "DQ 174" a fim de disfarçar a sua natureza. O tratamento continuou durante cinco dias.

O diflunisal provou ser superior ao ASA, causou menos efeitos secundários gástricos, e teve de ser suspenso menos vezes durante o tempo de estudo. Apresentava também a vantagem de ser administrado duas vezes por dia. A dose foi tantas vezes de 250 mg duas vezes/dia como de 500 mg duas vezes/dia. O diflunisal tem, portanto, óbvias vantagens sobre o ASA como um analgésico para uso em clínica geral.

Diflunisal: Long-term Efficacy and Safety in Geriatric Patients

D. C. GENGOS, A. ANDREW, W. F. HOFFMAN and A. R. RHYMER

*Merck Sharp & Dohme Research Laboratories,
Rahway, New Jersey, USA*

Diflunisal is a new prostaglandin synthetase (PGS) inhibitor which has been evaluated as an analgesic and was introduced into clinical practice in 1978.

The structural formula of diflunisal is illustrated in Fig. 1. It is a nonacetylated, difluorophenyl derivative of salicylic acid and is distinguished from acetylsalicylic acid (ASA) by chemical, metabolic, biological and pharmacokinetic differences (Hannah et al., 1977; Kuehl and Egan, 1978; Tempero et al., 1977). Diflunisal is a stable molecule and is not metabolized to salicylic acid.

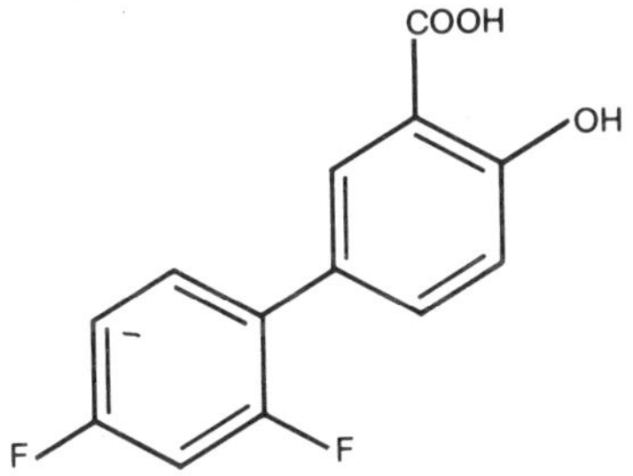

Figure 1. Structural formulae of diflunisal

In the studies which were completed to establish the analgesic effectiveness and safety of diflunisal, a series of surgical models was used to evaluate single dose and multiple dose short-term therapy in acute pain (Van Winzum and Rodda, 1977; Honig, 1978); musculoskeletal trauma to evaluate therapy in pain of intermediate duration (Barran, 1978); and the painful symptoms of chronic osteoarthritis (joint pain, night pain, inactivity stiffness, etc) in order to evaluate long-term safety and maintained efficacy (Andrew et al., 1977; Van Winzum et al., 1978). In these studies diflunisal was compared with acetylsalicylic acid, glafenine, phenylbutazone and ibuprofen. In subsequent studies diflunisal has been compared with a large number of

Diflunisal: Royal Society of Medicine International Congress and Symposium Series No. 6, published jointly by Academic Press Inc. (London) Ltd., and the Royal Society of Medicine.

analgesics and other PGS inhibitors in a broad range of clinical circumstances for the treatment of pain of acute and intermediate duration. This report deals with the long-term treatment with diflunisal of patients 65 years of age and over.

Patients and Methods

For long-term evaluation of pain relief and safety, chronic osteoarthritis was chosen as the model and 695 patients were entered into multi-clinic studies comparing diflunisal with ASA for 3 months using double-blind methodology with subsequent extensions for many patients to either 6 or 12 months of therapy. Of the patients entering these studies, 281 were 65 years of age and over.

Patients entered into this programme were those with a definite diagnosis of osteoarthritis characterized by pain (aggravated by active or passive movement, weight bearing and relieved by rest), night pain, inactivity stiffness, and limitation of passive motion of the affected joints. Patients with serious complicated diseases or other forms of arthritis were excluded. The concurrent administration of systemic steroidal or nonsteroidal anti-inflammatory agents, barbiturates, supplemental ASA or other analgesic drugs was forbidden. Physical therapy begun before the study could be continued unchanged, but no physical therapy was to be introduced during the study.

Patients were randomly assigned to receive 250 mg of diflunisal b.i.d. or 500 mg of ASA q.i.d. Therapy commenced when pain recurred after withdrawal of previous therapy or 7 days after the withdrawal. The study was double-blind with each patient receiving medication four times daily with the group treated with diflunisal having active tablets twice only (in the morning and in the evening). Dosage could be increased after one week so that the patients receiving diflunisal could have a maximum daily dosage of 750 mg; for those being treated with ASA, the maximum daily dose was 3000 mg. The investigators were advised not to increase dosage unless the clinical response to the initial dose was unsatisfactory. At the end of the double-blind period of the study, patients were invited to continue on their established drug in an open-label fashion for extensions up to one year. Not all of the investigators continued into each extension period so that the number of patients concluding one study period and extending into the next is not the same.

Patients were examined at the end of the withdrawal period and immediately before administration of the test drug to provide baseline evaluation of their pain symptoms. The efficacy criteria involved evaluation of both subjective and objective variables. Pain on weight bearing and night pain were rated on a 5-point scale with strictly defined categories ranging from absence of pain to pain that was totally disabling or seriously interfered with sleep. Inactivity stiffness was measured as the time necessary to gain appreciable improvement after inactivity. An overall assessment of therapeutic response was made by the patient and the investigator each using a 5-point scale.

Side effects were elicited from patients at each visit by discussing with them their general well being and asking whether they had any complaints; the investigator did not itemize specific side effects by direct questioning. Laboratory tests were assayed to detect possible effects on renal, hepatic or haemopoietic function.

Results

This multiclinic study involved 281 patients 65 years of age and over. Of this total 150 received treatment with diflunisal 131 received treatment with ASA. The charac-

Table 1

Sex by treatment group

	Diflunisal		ASA	
Age	Male	Female	Male	Female
65–69	20	60	23	47
70–74	15	49	15	42
Over 75	—	6	—	4
SUBTOTAL	35	115	38	93
TOTALS	150		131	

teristics of these patients in terms of age, sex and distribution to treatment groups is shown in Table 1.

The register of patients entering the programme in terms of those completing each study period and then discontinuing therapy during any study period are shown in Table 2.

Efficacy

Efficacy evaluation using relief of pain at night and on weight bearing, relief of inactivity stiffness, patients' assessment of overall relief and investigators' assessment of therapeutic effects are shown in Tables 3, 4, 5, 6 and 7. Not all of the patients were assessed for every parameter at the end of each study period so that the cohort groups for each parameter differs and in no case is it the same as the number of patients completing each segment of the study.

Freedom from night pain or persistence of only slight pain at night was recorded by 88% of the patients treated with diflunisal at 3 months. This compares with 45% of the patients at the start of the study who were free of night pain or only slightly bothered by it. This high percentage of patients who had relief of night pain was well

Table 2

Patients entering and completing each study period

	0–12 weeks		13–24 weeks		25–48 weeks	
	Diflunisal	ASA	Diflunisal	ASA	Diflunisal	ASA
Entered	150	131	78	49	43	19
Completed	120	86	71	42	34	12
Discontinuing	30	45	7	7	9	7

Percent of patients dropping out from 0–12 weeks higher for ASA ($P<0.01$).

Table 3

Relief of night pain

Treatment	Diflunisal				ASA			
Weeks on treatment	Baseline	0–12	13–24	25–48	Baseline	0–12	13–24	25–48
Number of patients evaluated	150	108	67	40	131	83	38	14
Rating	Percent				Percent			
1	14	69	66	74	27	65	68	57
2	31	19	24	24	23	24	16	36
3	24	8	7	0	29	7	13	0
4	25	3	3	2	16	4	3	0
5	6	1	0	0	5	0	0	7

1. no pain; 2. bothered some by pain; 3. bothered a lot by pain; 4. bothered terribly by pain; 5. worst possible pain.

maintained throughout the studies to one year (90% at 6 months and 98% at 1 year) (Table 3).

In the ASA group, 89% were free of night pain or only slightly bothered by it at 3 months compared with 50% at entry and this measure of relief was also maintained (84% at 6 months and 93% at one year) (Table 3).

Pain on weight bearing, which is in effect a measure of pain occurring throughout the day, persisted at a level rated as moderate to severe or severe in only 13% of the patients treated with diflunisal which compares with a figure of 60% of the patients with this degree of pain at entry. On the other hand, 62% were free of pain or complained of only mild pain at 3 months compared with 13% of the patients who were free of pain or had only mild pain at entry. At 6 months, 57% of patients were free of pain or had only mild pain, while at one year, the figure was 75% (Table 4).

Table 4

Relief of weight-bearing pain

Treatment	Diflunisal				ASA			
Weeks on treatment	Baseline	0–12	13–24	25–48	Baseline	0–12	13–24	25–48
Number of patients treated	150	115	68	40	131	81	38	14
Rating	Percent				Percent			
No pain	1	16	26	27	1	15	21	29
Mild pain	12	46	31	48	21	45	53	36
Mod. pain	27	25	28	20	30	25	16	14
Mod./severe pain	46	10	15	5	38	14	10	14
Severe pain	14	3	0	0	10	1	0	7

In the patients treated with ASA, 60% were either free of pain or had only mild pain at 3 months compared with 22% at entry, 74% at 6 months and 65% at one year. At entry, 48% of patients had pain which they rated at moderately severe to severe and at 3 months this was reduced to 15% of the patients; at 6 months, it was 10% and at one year, 21% (only 3 patients of 14) (Table 4).

Inactivity stiffness was measured in minutes required to be able to resume free activity. In the group treated with diflunisal, 85% of the patients at 3 months had only 5 min or less of stiffness compared with 44% with this short time of disability at entry to the study. At 6 months, 84% required only 5 min or less to recover from inactivity, and at 12 months, the figure was 92% (Table 5).

In the group treated with ASA, at entry 52% had inactivity stiffness requiring 5 min or less for recovery and at 3 months, 71% recovered in 5 min or less, while at 6 months and one year, the figures were 76% and 57% (Table 5).

Overall relief of symptoms was assessed by patients who were asked to rate the response afforded by their therapy on a 5-point scale. In the group treated with

Table 5

Relief of inactivity stiffness

Treatment	Diflunisal				ASA			
Weeks on treatment	Baseline	0–12	13–24	25–48	Baseline	0–12	13–24	25–48
Number of patients treated	150	112	68	38	131	84	37	14
Duration (Min)		Percent				Percent		
0	9	34	44	34	11	29	41	21
1–5	35	51	40	58	41	42	35	36
6–15	21	11	12	8	22	14	16	8
16–30	8	3	2	0	7	8	5	14
>30	27	1	2	0	19	7	3	21

Diflunisal superior to ASA during weeks 0–12 and 25–48 ($P<0.05$).

Table 6

Patient's assessment of overall relief

Treatment	Diflunisal			ASA		
Weeks on treatment	0–12	13–24	25–48	0–12	13–24	25–48
Number of patients treated	115	70	40	86	38	14
Rating		Percent			Percent	
None	4	1	0	6	0	14
Poor	11	6	10	14	13	7
Fair	21	21	10	23	32	7
Good	41	39	40	45	26	43
Excellent	23	33	40	12	29	29

diflunisal, 64% rated the therapy as excellent or good at 3 months, 72% at 6 months and 80% at one year (Table 6).

In the ASA group, 57% rated their overall relief as good or excellent at 3 months, 55% at 6 months and 72% at one year (Table 6).

Therapeutic effect was assessed by the investigators also using a 5-point scale, and in the group treated with diflunisal, 60% were assessed as having a good or excellent result at 3 months, 72% at 6 months and 86% at one year. For the patients treated with ASA, 62% were rated as having had a good or excellent therapeutic response at 3 months; 52% at 6 months and 75% at one year (Table 7).

Unsatisfactory therapeutic response was a cause for some patients dropping out in each period of the study. In the first 3 months, 8 patients, representing 5·3% of the 150 patients starting the study and treated with diflunisal, dropped out for this reason compared with 14 of the ASA group which is 10·7% of the 131 starting therapy. During the 3- to 6-month period, four of the patients treated with diflunisal dropped out (5%) because of ineffective therapy and a further 2 (4·6%) dropped out during the 6-month to one year period. In the ASA group, no patient dropped out in the 3- to 6-month period and one (5·2%) dropped out between 6 months and one year (Table 8).

Table 7

Investigator's assessment of therapeutic effect

Treatment	Diflunisal			ASA		
Weeks on treatment	0–12	13–24	25–48	0–12	13–24	25–48
Number of patients treated	119	72	42	86	40	16
Rating	Percent			Percent		
None	5	3	0	5	0	13
Poor	13	4	4	17	13	6
Fair	22	21	10	16	35	6
Good	38	40	48	48	17	44
Excellent	22	32	38	14	35	31

Diflunisal superior to ASA at weeks 13–24 ($P<0.05$).

Table 8

Patients discontinuing therapy

Treatment	Diflunisal	ASA	Diflunisal	ASA	Diflunisal	ASA
Weeks on treatment	0–12		13–24		25–48	
Number of patients treated	150	131	78	49	43	19
	Percentages					
Clinical side effect	8·6	19	0	6	4·6	10·5
Abnormal laboratory value	0·6	0	0	2	0	0
Unsatisfactory therapeutic Resp.	5·3	10·7	5	0	4·6	5·2
Not treatment related	5·3	4·6	3·8	6	11·6	21

Percent of patients discontinuing because of side effects significantly fewer for diflunisal than ASA ($P<0.05$).

Tolerance and safety

Of the 150 patients who started therapy with diflunisal, 13 patients (8·6%) dropped out because of the occurrence of one or more side-effects in the first 3 months. Of the 131 patients who started therapy with ASA, 25 (19%) dropped out because of side-effects occurring in the first 3 months. During the period between the third and sixth month, no patients treated with diflunisal dropped out, while 6% (3 of 49) in the ASA group dropped out. In the period between the sixth and twelfth month of therapy, two of 43 (4·6%) of the patients treated with diflunisal dropped out because of side effects and two of 19 (10·5%) of the ASA patients also dropped out (Table 8). The percentage of patients who dropped out for other causes unrelated to therapy is also shown in Table 8. Only two patients dropped out of the studies because of abnormal laboratory values. One patient treated with diflunisal had transient elevations of serum alkaline phosphatase and SGOT levels during the first 3 months of therapy. During the second 3 months of therapy, one patient treated with ASA had an elevated white blood count. The types of side-effects which caused patients to discontinue therapy are shown in Table 9. Overall side-effects which were drug-related were otherwise

Table 9
Number of patients discontinuing because of side-effects

Treatment	Diflunisal	ASA	Diflunisal	ASA	Diflunisal	ASA
Cohort	150	131	78	49	43	19
Discontinued	13	25	0	3	2	2
Percentage	8·6	19·1	—	6	4·6	10·5
Type of side effect						
G.I.						
upper	12	28	—	3	2	1
lower	1	1	—	—	—	—
CNS						
vertigo	—	1	—	—	—	—
tinnitus	—	—	—	1	—	1
other	1	5	—	—	—	—
CVS	1	2	—	—	—	—
Respiratory	2	—	—	—	1	—
Cutaneous	1	5	—	—	—	1
Haematologic	—	4	—	—	—	—
Other	—	1	—	2	—	—

Table 10
Percent of patients reporting drug-related clinical side-effects

Treatment	Diflunisal			ASA		
Weeks of treatment	0–12	13–24	25–48	0–12	13–24	25–48
Number of patients evaluated for safety	150	78	43	131	49	19
Percent reporting side effects	19	4	0	48	30	5

Incidence of side effects significantly lower for diflunisal than for ASA weeks 0–12 and 13–25 ($P<0.05$).

mild. Gastrointestinal and central nervous system side-effects occurred in greater number and more frequently in patients treated with ASA than with diflunisal. The majority of these side-effects occured in the first 3 months of therapy and the percentage of patients involved is shown in Table 10.

Discussion

Diflunisal has analgesic properties similar to those of acetylsalicylic acid but is considerably more potent and exerts its effect over a longer period of time so that it is prescribed by a twice-a-day schedule. Salicylates are now recognized as prostaglandin synthetase inhibitors and in analgesic terms are classified as peripheral analgesics.

Pain is a major symptom of disease and pain relief is the major objective of much treatment. Analgesics are prescribed both for short-term and long-term use and, in the latter case, patients often exercise considerable latitude in their daily dose schedules.

Pain is a subjective phenomenon and the simplest method of measuring it is to have the sufferers rate their perception of pain or its relief in subjective terms.

In the studies reported diflunisal was rated as effective as ASA in the relief of chronic pain of osteoarthritis but achieved this equality in analgesia by a twice-a-day dose schedule compared with the usual 3 to 4 times a day schedule required for effective pain relief with ASA. It is notable that this twice-a-day schedule provided effective relief of pain both throughout the day and night.

In reviewing the experience of patients 65 years and over, it was found that these patients tolerated diflunisal better than they did ASA. Fewer patients discontinued treatment because of ineffective therapy or intolerance and the good response to therapy was maintained throughout the full year of therapy in those groups of patients continuing treatment beyond 3 and 6 months.

Conclusions

Diflunisal at doses up to 750 mg per day was used to treat the painful symptoms of chronic osteoarthritis in a group of 281 patients aged 65 years and over for periods up to one year. Analgesic effectiveness and safety of tolerance of diflunisal was compared with that of ASA.

Diflunisal given on a twice-a-day dose schedule and at doses which were a quarter those of ASA was found to be equianalgesic in terms of the relief of weight bearing pain throughout the day and pain throughout the night. Diflunisal was better tolerated than ASA and is proposed as an analgesic agent which is suitable for use in geriatric patients for relief of pain whether for short-term or prolonged therapy.

References

Andrew, A., Rodda, B., Verhaest, L., and Van Winzum, C. (1977). *Br. J. Clin. Pharmac.* **4**, 455.
Barran, J. (1978). *Clin. Ther.* **1**, (Supp. A), 43.
Hannah, J., Ruyle, W. V., Jones, H., Matzuk, A. R., Kelly, K. W., Witzel, B. E., Holtz, W. J., Houser, R. W., Shen, T. Y. and Sarett, L. H. (1977). *Br. J. Clin. Pharmac.* **4**, 75.

Honig, W. J. (1978). "Diflunisal in Clinical Practice", Futura Press, New York.
Kuehl, F. A., and Egan R. W. (1978). "Diflunisal in Clinical Practice", Futura Press, New York.
Tempero, K. F., Cirillo, V. J. and Steelman, S. L. (1977). *Br. J. Clin. Pharmac.* **4**, 315.
Van Winzum, C. and Rodda, B. (1977). *Br. J. Clin. Pharmac.* **4**, 395.
Van Winzum, C., Cook, T., Verhaest, L., and Andrew, A. (1978). "Diflunisal in Clinical Practice", Futura Press, New York.

Summary

In studies to establish the analgesic effectiveness and safety of diflunisal a series of surgical models was used to evaluate single dose and multiple dose short-term therapy; musculoskeletal trauma to evaluate therapy of intermediate duration; and the painful symptoms of chronic osteoarthritis (joint pain, night pain, inactivity stiffness, etc.) to evaluate long-term safety and maintained efficacy of 800 patients with osteoarthritis who entered two double-blind studies comparing diflunisal with ASA and ibuprofen for periods of 3–12 months, 304 were 65 years of age and over and the experiences of these patients are the subject of this report. A definite diagnosis of active osteoarthritis of the hip or knee was required for entry into the study. The patients had pain which was aggravated by active motion and at least partially relieved by rest; inactivity stiffness and at least grade 2 changes on X-ray examination. Following a withdrawal of previous therapy for periods up to 7 days patients were randomly assigned to receive 250 mg of diflunisal b.i.d. or 500 mg of ASA q.i.d. or 800 mg ibuprofen daily by a t.i.d. schedule. Dosage could be increased after 1 week so that the patients receiving diflunisal reached a daily dose of 3000 mg and the ibuprofen group received up to 1200 mg/day. Diflunisal was highly effective in the relief of painful symptoms of chronic arthritis (joint pain, night pain, inactivity stiffness, etc.) and in most parameters was better than the comparative agents. Diflunisal was well tolerated with fewer overall side-effects than the comparative agents both in numbers of patients reporting side-effects and the types of side-effects.

Zusammenfassung

In Studien zur Bestimmung der analgesischen Wirksamkeit und Sicherheit von Diflunisal wurde eine Reihe chirurgischer Modelle benutzt, um die kurzfristige Einfach- und Mehrfachdosen-Therapie auszuwerten; Skelettmuskulaturtrauma zur Auswertung der Therapie von Zwischendauer, und die schmerzhaften Symptome von chronischer Osteoarthritis (Gelenkschmerz, Nachtschmerz, durch Untätigkeit bedingte Steifigkeit usw.) zur Auswertung der langfristigen Sicherheit und Dauerwirksamkeit. Von 800 Patienten mit Osteoarthritis, die sich zu zwei doppelt blinden Studien zur Verfügung stellten, in denen Diflunisal und Ibuprofen für Zeiträume von 3–12 Monaten verglichen wurden, waren 304 65 Jahre alt und älter, und die Erfahrungen dieser Patienten sind Gegenstand dieses Berichtes. Für die Teilnahme an der Studie war eine eindeutige Diagnose von aktiver Osteoarthritis der Hüfte oder des Knies erforderlich. Die Patienten litten Schmerzen, die durch aktive Bewegung noch erhöht wurden und durch Ruhe zumindest teilweise gelindert wurden; durch Untätigkeit bedingte Steifigkeit und Änderungen von zumindest Stufe 2 bei der Röntgenuntersuchung. Nach einem Zurückziehen der früheren Therapie für Zeiträume bis zu sieben Tagen wurden Patienten wahllos zugeteilt, um 250 mg Diflunisal zweimal tgl. oder 500 mg ASA viermal tgl. oder 800 mg Ibuprofen dreimal täglich zu erhalten. Die Dosierung konnte nach einer Woche erhöht werden, so daß Diflunisal erhaltende Patienten eine Tagesdosis von 3000 mg erreichten und die Ibuprofen-Gruppe bis zu 1200 mg/Tag erheilt.

Diflunisal erwies sich in der Linderung der schmerzhaften Symptome chronischer Arthritis (Gelenkschmerz, Nachtschmerz, durch Unätitigkeit bedingte Steifigkeit usw.) als äußerst wirksam und war in den meisten Parametern besser als die Vergleichsmittel. Diflunisal wurde gut vertragen und brachte weniger Gesamtnebenwirkungen als die Vergleichsmittel sowohl in der Anzahl von Patienten, die Nebenwirkungen meldeten, als auch in der Art der Nebenwirkungen.

Résumé

Dans des études destinées à établir l'efficacité et l'innocuité du diflunisal, on utilise une série de modèles chirurgicaux pour évaluer le traitement à court terme à dose unique et à doses multiples, le trauma musculo-squelettique pour évaluer le traitement de moyenne durée, et les symptômes douloureux de l'ostéoarthrite chronique (douleurs dans les articulations, douleurs nocturnes, raideur due à l'inactivité, etc.) pour évaluer l'innocuité à long terme et la persistance de l'efficacité. 800 malades souffrant d'ostéoarthrite ont fait l'objet de deux études de comparaison du diflunisal avec l'acide acétylsalicylique et l'ibuprofène pendant des périodes de 3 à 12 mois. 304 d'entre eux avaient 65 ans et plus, et le présent compte-rendu est consacré aux résultats obtenus sur ces malades. Un diagnostic net d'ostéoarthrite active de la hanche ou du genou était exigé. Les douleurs des malades étaient aggravées par le mouvement actif et au moins partiellement soulagées par le repos; ils présentaient de la raideur due à l'inactivité et des changements de catégorie 2 au moins dans l'examen aux rayons X. Après un arrêt du traitement précédent pendant 1 à 7 jours, les malades etaient désignés au hasard pour recevoir 250 mg de diflunisal deux fois par jour ou 500 mg d'acide acétylsalicylique quatre fois par jour ou 800 mg d'ibuprofène par jour (en trois fois). Les doses pouvaient être accrues au bout d'une semaine, de sorte que les malades pouvaient recevoir une dose journalière de 3000 mg de diflunisal ou de 1200 mg d'ibuprofène.

Le diflunisal est très efficace pour soulager les symptômes douloureux de l'arthrite chronique (douleurs dans les articulations, douleurs nocturnes, raideur due à l'inactivité, etc.) et se montre supérieur aux deux autres médicaments à presque tous les égards. Le diflunisal est bien toléré, avec moins d'effets secondaires que les deux autres médicaments (moins de malades signalant des effets secondaires et effets secondaires plus légers).

Sommario

In studi per stabilire l'efficacia analgesica e la sicurezza del diflunisal in terapia a breve termine con somministrazione a dosi uniche o multiple, si impiegò una serie di modelli chirurgici; trauma muscolo-scheletrici per il medio termine, e sindromi dolorose da osteoartrite cronica (anchilosi, dolori notturni, rigiditàd a inattività, ecc.) per il lungo termine. Di 800 pazienti affetti da osteoartrite facenti parte di due studi "double-blind" con cui si raffrontò il diflunisal con l'acido acetilsalicilico e l'ibuprofene per un periodo di 3–12 mesi, 300 erano di età superiore o uguale a 65 anni. Le esperienze avute con questi pazienti formano l'oggetto di questa relazione. Nei gruppi di studio si ammisero pazienti con osteoartrite attiva dell'anca o ginocchio. I pazienti presentavano dolori che si aggravavano con il movimento dell'articolazione e si alleviavano, almeno in parte, con il riposo, nonchè rigidità da inattività e, almeno, cambiamenti di secondo grado all'esame radiografico. Dopo averli tolti dalla cura precedente per periodi di fino a 7 giorni, i pazienti vennero assegnati casualmente a 3 gruppi: diflunisal in dosi da 250 mg due volte al giorno; acido acetilsalicilico in dosi da 500 mg quattro volte al giorno; e ibuprofene in dosi da 800 mg tre volte al giorno. Si poterono aumentare le dosi giornaliere fino a 3000 mg per il diflunisal e fino a 1200 mg per l'ibuprofene dopo 1 settimana dell' inizio del trattamento.

Il diflunisal si rivelò molto efficace nella terapia del dolore da artriti croniche (anchilosi, dolori notturni, rigidità da inattività, ecc.) e, nella maggior parte dei parametri, migliore degli altri farmaci. Il diflunisal fu ben tollerato e presentò globalmente minori effetti secondari a confronto degli altri farmaci, sia per quanto riguarda il tipo di effetto secondario che il numero dei pazienti da essi affetti.

Resumen

Para establecer la eficacia analgésica y la seguridad del diflunisal, se utilizaron una serie de modelos quirúrgicos que permitieran evaluar la terapia a corto plazo de dosis única y múltiples, así como el trauma musculoesquelético para evaluar la terapia de duración intermedia y el síndrome doloroso de la artrosis crónica (dolor articular, dolor nocturno, rigidez por inactividad) para evaluar la seguridad a largo plazo y la eficacia sostenida. Ochocientos pacientes con artrosis participaron en dos estudios a doble ciego, comparando el diflunisal con el AAS y el ibuprofen por periodos de 3 a 12 meses. De éstos, 304 eran de 65 o más años y las experiencias con este grupo se relatan en este informe. Para entrar en el estudio se requería un diagnóstico definitivo de artrosis activa de cadera o rodilla. Los pacientes tenían dolor que se acentuaba con la actividad y mejoraba algo con el reposo; rigidez por inactividad y cambios radiográficos de grado 2 por lo menos. Después de interrumpir la terapia anterior por periodos de 1 a 7 días, los pacientes recibieron al azar 250 mg de diflunisal dos veces por día o 500 mg de AAS cuatro veces por día u 800 mg de ibuprofen tres veces por día. La dosis podía aumentarse luego de una semana, de manera que los pacientes con diflunisal alcanzasen una dosis diaria de 3000 mg y el grupo de ibuprofen hasta 1200 mg por día. El diflunisal demostró ser muy eficaz en el alivio de los síntomas dolorosos de la artritis crónica (dolor articular, dolor nocturno, rigidez por inactividad, etc.) y mejor que los agentes de comparación en la mayoría de los parámetros. El diflunisal se toleró bien con menos efectos secundarios que los agentes de comparación, tanto en el número de pacientes que comunicaron efectos secundarios como en los tipos de tales efectos.

Sumário

Em estudos designados a estabelecer a eficácia analgésica e grau de segurança do diflunisal, foi usada uma série de casos cirúrgicos para avaliar a terapia a curto-prazo em dose única e doses múltiplas; trauma músculo-esquelético para avaliar terapia de duração intermédia; e os sintomas dolorosos de osteo-artrite crónica (dores articulares, dores nocturnas, rigidez de inactividade, etc.) para avaliar o grau de segurança a longo-prazo e a persistência de eficácia. Dos 800 doentes com osteo-artrite que participaram em dois estudos duplamente às cegas comparando o diflunisal com o ASA e o ibuprofen durante períodos de 3-12 meses, 304 tinham 65 anos de idade ou mais, e as experiências destes doentes constituem o tema deste relatório. Para entrar neste estudo era requerido um diagnóstico definitivo de osteo-artrite activa da anca ou joelho. Os doentes tinham dores que se intensificavam ao movimento activo e eram aliviadas, pelo menos parcialmente, pelo repouso; tinham também rigidez de inactividade e alterações, pelo menos do segundo grau, ao exame radiográfico. Após suspensão de qualquer terapêutica anterior, durante períodos de até sete dias, os doentes foram repartidos ao acaso por três grupos de tratamento, a saber: 250 mg de diflunisal 2 vezes/dia; ou 500 mg de ASA 4 vezes/dia; ou 800 mg de ibuprofen diàriamente (repartido em três doses). A dose podia ser aumentada ao fim de uma semana, de modo que os doentes tratados com diflunisal atingiram uma dose diária de 3.000 mg, e o grupo ibuprofen chegou a uma dose de 1200 mg/dia. O diflunisal foi extremamente eficaz no alívio de sintomas dolorosos de artrite crónica (dores articulares, dores nocturnas, rigidez de inactividade, etc.) e na maioria dos parâmetros foi melhor do que os agentes de comparação. A tolerância ao diflunisal foi boa produzindo, de maneira global, menos efeitos secundários do que os agentes de comparação, e isto tanto no que respeita ao número de doentes com queixas de efeitos secundários como quanto aos tipos de tais efeitos.

The Current Status of Diflunisal

E. C. HUSKISSON

St Bartholomew's Hospital, London, England

It is clear that diflunisal is a very different compound from its illustrious ancestor, aspirin, from which it was derived by a piece of brilliant molecular manipulation. First it has a long half-life which allows twice daily administration and perhaps provides pain relief throughout the night. Second it is a little more effective than aspirin, perhaps the result of fluorination of the aspirin molecule. Third it causes much fewer gastric side-effects than aspirin, does not cause tinnitus and deafness and may be safer than aspirin. Diflunisal does not have the same effect on platelets as aspirin; does not cause gastric microbleeding; has not caused a metabolic acidosis in the few overdoses so far seen and does not cause the hepatic changes which occasionally occur with aspirin. The safety and tolerance of the compound may be related to the removal of acetyl group from aspirin.

In this publication we have seen evidence that diflunisal is effective in low back pain, osteoarthritis, post-operative pain, dental pain, sprains and strains, rheumatoid arthritis and cancer pain. It clearly has a prolonged action and it has been shown to be superior over 8 h to the shorter acting analgesics. It appears that the dose required is between 250–500 mg b.i.d. and one would expect that the larger doses would be required in conditions like rheumatoid arthritis.

We have seen that diflunisal is as effective as the combination of dextropropoxyphene and paracetamol (Distalgesic, Darvocet N) which is very widely used as a simple analgesic. It is also equivalent to oral pentazocine. We have seen a comparison with oxyphenbutazone which suggested that diflunisal may be a little superior. We have seen studies comparing it with codeine phosphate, dextropropoxyphene and glafenine again showing that diflunisal is superior. We have seen many comparisons with aspirin in different indications all showing the diflunisal is superior. This has been shown in osteoarthritis, rheumatoid arthritis and also in the wide variety of pains which are seen in general practice.

We have heard very little about side-effects perhaps because there are not many. In my experience there have been a few cases of nausea and various other gastro-intestinal complaints including diarrhoea but it is clear from the papers in this publication that the overall incidence of side-effects with this drug is extremely low. Compared to aspirin there are less gastric side effects and tinnitus and deafness have not been a problem at doses so far used. Evidence has been presented that this is a very safe drug. It does not appear to have any important interactions and can be given with warfarin. Some care should be taken when diflunisal is started in a patient taking warfarin with daily measurement of prothrombin time for the first few days. Diflunisal does not cause occult gastrointestinal bleeding and it is nice to know that you can relieve pain and take alcohol as well. Overdosage has been discussed and is clearly very important for a drug which is to be widely used as an analgesic and will be left in patients' bathroom cupboards. Many of the drugs which are used as analgesics are really rather dangerous in overdose but preliminary experiences suggest that diflunisal may be safer in this respect.

Experiences reported in this symposium suggest that diflunisal will be a useful addition to the drugs already available for the treatment of pain. I imagine that because of its prolonged action it will be particularly useful for patients who require either a course of treatment or chronic administration of an analgesic. For those requiring a course I imagine it will be particularly useful in the treatment of low back pain, sprains and strains and injuries of various sorts— illnesses which last a few days or weeks. For chronic administration it will be useful in various chronic arthritic diseases and in patients with cancer pain.

Der gegenwartige Status von Diflunisal

E. C. HUSKISSON

St Bartholomew's Hospital, London, England

Es ist klar, daß Diflunisal eine von seinem illustren Vorgänger, Aspirin, von dem es durch ein Stück brillianter molekularer Manipulation hergeleitet wurde, stark abweichende Zusammensetzung ist. Erstens hat es eine Halbwertzeit, die eine Verabreichung zweimal täglich gestattet und wahrscheinlich eine Schmerzlinderung während der ganzen Nacht vorsieht. Zweitens ist es etwas wirksamer als Aspirin—wahrscheinlich das Ergebnis der Fluorination des Aspirin-Moleküls. Drittens verursacht es weniger gastrische Nebenwirkungen als Aspirin, verursacht kein Ohrenklingen und keine Taubheit und kann sicherer sein als Aspirin. Diflunisal hat nicht dieselbe Wirkung auf Blutplättchen wie Aspirin, verursacht keine gastrische Mikroblutung, hat in den bisher gesehenen wenigen Überdosen keine Stoffwechselazidose und verursacht nicht die hepatischen Veränderungen, wie sie gelegentlich bei Aspirin auftreten. Die Sicherheit und Toleranz der Zusammensetzung kann mit der Entfernung der Azetylgruppe aus Aspirin in Beziehung gesetzt werden.

In diesem Symposium haben wir den Beweis dafür gesehen, daß Diflunisal in tiefliegendem Rückenschmerz, Osteoarthritis, post-operativem Schmerz, Zahnschmerz, Verstauchungen und Zerrungen, rheumaartiger Arthritis und Krebsschmerz wirksam ist. Es hat eindeutig eine Langzeitwirkung, und es wurde nachgewiesen, daß es über acht Stunden den kürzer wirkenden schmerzlindernden Mitteln überlegen ist. Es scheint so, als ob die benötigte Dosis zwischen 250-500 mg zweimal täglich beträgt, und man würde erwarten, daß die größeren Dosen in Zuständen wie rheumaartiger Arthritis benötigt würden.

Wir haben gesehen, daß Diflunisal ebenso wirksam ist wie die Kombination von Dextropropoxyphen und Paracetamol (Distalgetikum, Darvocet N), die als einfaches Analgetikum weitgehend benutzt wird. Es ist ebenfalls gleichwertig mit Pentazocine. Wir haben einen Vergleich mit Oxyphenbutazon gesehen, der andeutete, daß Diflunisal etwas überlegen sein kann. Wir haben Studien gesehen, in denen es mit Kodeinphosphat, Dextropropoxyphen und Glafenin vergleicht wird, und welche wiederum zeigen, daß Diflunisal überlegen ist. Wir haben ziemlich viele Vergleiche mit Aspirin in verschiedenen Indikationen gesehen, die sämtlich ausweisen, daß Diflunisal überlegen ist. Das wurde in Osteoarthritis, rheumaartiger Arthritis sowie ebenfalls in einer Vielzahl von Schmerzen nachgewiesen, die man in der Allgemeinpraxis verzeichnet.

Wir haben sehr wenig über Nebenwirkungen gehört—wahrscheinlich deshalb,

---

Diflusinal: Royal Society of Medicine International Congress and Symposium Series No. 6, published jointly by Academic Press Inc. (London) Ltd., and the Royal Society of Medicine.

weil es nicht viele gibt. Nach meiner eigenen Erfahrung hat es einige wenige Fälle von Erbrechen und verschiedene andere gastrointestinale Beschwerden einschließlich Diarrhöe gegeben, jedoch ist es anhand der Abhandlungen in diesem Symposium klar, daß das Gesamtauftreten von Nebenwirkungen bei dieser Droge äußerst selten ist. Im Vergleich zu Aspirin gibt es weniger gastrische Nebenwirkungen, und Ohrenklingen und Taubheit sind bei den bisher benutzten Dosen kein Problem gewesen. Es wurde der Nachweis erbracht, daß es eine äußerst sichere Droge ist. Es scheint keinerlei bedeutende Wechselwirkungen zu haben und kann mit Warfarin verabreicht werden. Eine gewisse Vorsicht ist geboten, wenn Diflunisal an einem Warfarin nehmenden Patienten erstmals benutzt wird; während der ersten Tage sind tägliche Messungen der Prothrombinzeit vorzunehmen. Diflunisal verursacht keine okkulte gastrointestinale Blutung, und es ist erfreulich zu wissen, daß man Schmerzen lindern und gleichzeitig Alkohol trinken kann. Die Überdosierung wurde ebenfalls besprochen und ist eindeutig sehr wichtig für eine Droge, die weitgehend als Analgetikum benutzt werden soll und in den Badezimmerschränken der Patienten gelassen wird. Viele der als schmerzlindernde Mittel verwendeten Drogen sind in Überdosen wirklich ziemlich gefährlich, jedoch deuten Voraberfahrungen an, daß Diflunisal in dieser Hinsicht sicherer sein kann.

Die in diesem Symposium berichteten Erfahrungen deuten an, daß Diflunisal eine nützliche Ergänzung der zur Behandlung von Schmerzen bereits verfügbaren Drogen sein wird. Ich kann mir vorstellen, daß es sich dank seiner Langzeitwirkung besonders für solche Patienten als nützlich erweisen wird, die entweder eines Heilverfahrens oder einer lange dauernden Verabreichung eines Analgetikums bedürfen. Für diejenigen, die eines Verfahrens bedürfen, wird es m.E. in der Behandlung von tief liegendem Rückenschmerz, Verstauchungen und Zerrungen sowie Verletzungen verschiedener Art—Krankheiten, die einige Tage oder Wochen dauern—besonders nützlich sein. Für die lange dauernde Verabreichung wird es sich in verschiedenen chronischen arthritischen Leiden und in Patienten mit Krebsschmerzen als nützlich erweisen.

Situation actuelle du diflunisal

E. C. HUSKISSON

St Bartholomew's Hospital, London, England

Il est manifeste que le diflunisal est un composé très différent de son illustre ancêtre, l'aspirine, dont il a été dérivé par une brillante manipulation moléculaire. En premier lieu, il a une longue période de demi-valeur, ce qui permet de l'administrer deux fois par jour et peut-être d'obtenir le soulagement de la douleur pendant la nuit. En second lieu, il est un peu plus efficace que l'aspirine, ce qui tient peut-être à la fluoration de la molécule d'aspirine. En troisième lieu, il produit beaucoup moins d'effets secondaires gatriques que ne produit pas de tintements d'oreilles ni de surdité, et est probablement plus sûr que l'aspirine. Le diflunisal n'a pas le même effet que l'aspirine sur les plaquettes du sang, ne produit pas de microhémorragie gastrique, n'a pas produit d'acidose métabolique dans les quelques cas de surdosage observés, et ne produit pas les modifications hépatiques qui ont parfois lieu avec l'aspirine. La sécurité et la tolérance du composé sont sans doute liées à l'élimination du groupe acétyle de l'aspirine.

Dans ce colloque, nous avons eu des preuves que le diflunisal est efficace envers le lumbago, l'ostéoarthrite, les douleurs post-opératoires, les douleurs dentaires, les foulures et élongations, l'arthrite rhumatismale et les douleurs du cancer. Il a manifestement une action prolongée et s'est montré supérieur sur une période de huit heures aux analgésiques à action plus brève. Il apparaît que la posologie requise est comprise entre 2×250 mg et 2×500 mg par jour; il est à prévoir que les doses maximales seront nécessaires dans des états tels que l'arthrite rhumatismale.

Nous avons vu que le diflunisal est aussi efficace que la combinaison de dextropropoxyphène et de paracétamol ("distalgésique", "darvocet N"), qui est très répandue comme analgésique simple. Il est aussi équivalent à la pentazocine. Nous avons vu une comparaison avec l'oxyphenbutazone qui paraît indiquer que le diflunisal est légèrement supérieur. Nous avons vu des études comparatives avec le phosphate de codéine, le dextropropoxyphène et la glafénine, qui montrent également la supériorité du diflunisal. Nous avons vu de nombreuses comparaisons avec l'aspirine dans des indications diverses, qui montrent toutes la supériorité du diflunisal, notamment dans l'ostéoarthrite, l'arthrite rhumatismale, ainsi que dans diverses douleurs rencontrées en médecine générale.

Nous avons très peu entendu parler d'effets secondaires, sans doute parce qu'il y en a peu. D'après mon expérience, il y a eu quelques cas de nausée et de vivers autres troubles gastro-intestinaux, dont la diarrhée, mais il est manifeste d'après ces exposés

---

Diflunisal: Royal Society of Medicine International Congress and Symposium Series No. 6, published jointly by Academic Press Inc. (London) Ltd., and the Royal Society of Medicine.

que la fréquence globale des effets secondaires dus à ce médicament est extrêmement faible. Par comparaison avec l'aspirine, il y a moins d'effets secondaires gastriques; les tintements d'oreilles et la surdité ne sont pas apparus jusqu'ici. Nous avons vu des preuves de l'innocuité de ce médicament. Il ne paraît pas avoir d'interactions importantes, et il peut être administré avec la warfarine. Il faut prendre quelques précautions quand on commence à administrer du diflunisal avec de la warfarine, en mesurant le temps de prothrombine pendant les quelques premiers jours. Le diflunisal ne produit pas d'hémorragie gastro-intestinale occulte, et il est agréable de savoir qu'on peut soulager la douleur et absorber de l'alcool. Le surdosage a été étudié: il a manifestement une grande importance pour un médicament destiné à être très utilisé comme analgésique et à être laissé dans les armoires de salle de bains des malades. Bien des médicaments utilisés comme analgésiques sont en réalité assez dangereux en surdose, mais les premières expériences paraissent indiquer que le diflunisal est assez peu dangereux à cet égard.

Les expériences rapportées dans ce colloque paraissent indiquer que le diflunisal sera un complément utile aux médicaments existants pour le traitement de la douleur. J'imagine qu'en raison de son action prolongée, il sera particulièrement utile pour les malades qui exigent soit un traitement prolongé, soit une administration chronique d'analgésique. Pour ceux qui exigent un traitement, j'imagine qu'il sera particulièrement utile dans le traitement du lumbago, des foulures et élongations et des lésions diverses, maladies qui durent quelques jours ou quelques mois. Pour l'administration chronique, il sera utile dans diverses maladies arthritiques chroniques et chez les malades souffrant de douleurs dues à un cancer.

La situazione attuale del Diflunisal

E. C. HUSKISSON
St Bartholomew's Hospital, London, England

E' evidente che il diflunisal è un composto molto differente dal suo illustre antenato, l'aspirina, dalla quale lo si è derivato mediante una brillante manipolazione molecolare. In primo luogo il diflunisal presenta un lungo periodo di dimezzamento, ciò che consente di limitare la somministrazione due volte al giorno e forse anche avere azione analgesica per tutta la notte. In secondo luogo è un poco più efficace dell'aspirina, forse per via della fluorinazione della molecola di quest'ultima. In terzo luogo causa minor effetti secondari gastrici dell'aspirina, non provoca ronzii auricolari nè sordità, e potrà essere di impiego più sicuro dell'aspirina. Il diflunisal non ha lo stesso effetto dell'aspirina sulle piastrine matiche, non causa microemorragie gastriche, non ha causato alcuna acidosi metabilica nei casi di dose eccessiva finora osservati, e non provoca i cambiementi epatici che si verificano di quando in quando con l'aspirina. La sicurezza e la tolleranza del composto si potranno collegare con l'asportazione del gruppo acetile dall'aspirina.

In questo simposio abbiamo visto prove dell'efficacia del diflunisal come analgesico in male di reni, osteoartrite, dolori postoperatori, mal di denti, distorsioni, artrite reumatoide e cancro. E' evidente che il diflunisal possiede un lungo tempo di azione che si è mostrato essere superiore di oltre 8 ore ad analgesici di durata più breve. A quanto sembra la dose richiesta va da 250 a 500 mg due volte al giorno e si prevedono dosi maggiori in casi come l'artrite reumatoide.

Abbiamo visto che il diflunisal è altrettanto efficace della combinazione destropropossifene/paracetamol (distalgesic, darvocet N) che è largamente impiegata come analgesico comune. E' pure equivalente alla pentazocina. Abbiamo visto una prova comparativa con l'ossifenbutazone dalla quale traspare che il diflunisal potrà essere un poco superiore. Abbiamo visto studi che lo mettono a raffronto con il fosfato di codeina, destropropossifene e glafcnina i quali mostrano pure la superiorità del diflunisal. Abbiamo visto molte prove comparative con l'aspirina in differenti situazioni, prove che tutte mostrano la superiorità del diflunisal. Lo si è mostrato nella osteoartrite, artrite reumatoide e pure nei numerosi tipi di algie che si presentano in medicina generale.

Abbiamo sentito parlare ben poco di effetti secondari forse perchè non ce ne sono stati molti. Personalmente ho incontrato solo alcuni casi di nausea e altri vari disturbi gastro-intestinali, compresa diarrea, però risulta evidente dai saggi presentati a questo simposio che con il diflunisal è molto bassa l'incidenza globale degli effetti secondari. A paragone dell'aspirina si hanno meno disturbi gastrici, e ronzio e sordità non hanno costituito un problema alle dosi finora impiegate. Le prove presentate dicono che si tratta di un medicamento molto sicuro. Non sembra che abbia alcuna importante interazione con altri farmaci e può venire somministrata assieme alla warfarina. Si dovrà fare una certa attenzione qualora si prescriva il diflunisal a pazienti in cura con warfarina, misurando giornalmente per i primi giorni il tempo di protrombina. Il diflunisal non dà luogo a emorragie gastro-intestinali occulte ed è rassicurante sapere che si può alleviare il dolore senza dover proibire gli alcolici. Si sono pure discussi gli effetti in caso di dosi eccessive, ciò che ovviamente è molto importante per un farmaco che sarà di uso comune come analgesico e quindi alla portata di mano del paziente. Molti dei farmaci impiegati come analgesici sono molto pericolosi se ingeriti in dosi eccessive, però le esperienze preliminari lasciano intendere che, a tale riguardo, il diflunisal possa essere sicuro.

Le esperienze rese note in questo simposio indicano che il diflunisal costituirà un'aggiunta utile ai farmaci già a disposizione per il trattamento delle algie. Grazie al suo effetto prolungato, penso che il diflunisal sia particolarmente utile per quei pazienti per i quali è necessaria una cura completa oppure la somministrazione cronica di un analgesico. Nel caso di cura, penso che il diflunisal sarà particolarmente utile nel trattamento di male di reni, distorsioni e lesioni e traumi di vario genere, infermità cioè che durano alcuni giorni o settimane. Nel caso della somministrazione cronica, sarà utile in varie affezioni croniche di natura artritica e in algie da cancro.

Situación actual del Diflunisal

E. C. HUSKISSON

St Bartholomew's Hospital, London, England

Es evidente que el diflunisal es un compuesto muy diferente de su ilustre antecesor, la aspirina, de la cual se derivó mediante una brillante manipulación molecular. En primer lugar, tiene una vida media prolongada que permite un régimen de dosificación de dos veces por día y quizá alivia el dolor toda la noche. En segundo lugar, es un poco más eficaz que la aspirina, quizá debido a la fluoración de la molécula de aspirina. En tercer lugar, tiene muchas menos repercusiones gástricas que la aspirina, no causa tinitus ni sordera y quizá sea más seguro que la aspirina. El diflunisal no tiene el mismo efecto plaquetario que la aspirina, ni causa microsangrado gástrico y tampoco produce acidosis metabólica en las pocas intoxicaciones hasta ahora observadas ni los cambios hepáticos que a veces ocurren con la aspirina.

En este simposio se han presentado pruebas de que el diflunisal es eficaz para el lumbago, la artrosis, el dolor post operatorio, el dolor de muelas, esguinces y desgarramientos, la artritis reumatoidea y los dolores del cáncer. Tiene una clara acción prolongada y ha mostrado ser superior en más de ocho horas a los analgésicos de acción corta. Parece ser que la dosis necesaria oscila entre los 250 mg y 500 mg por día y se supone que se necesitarán las dosis mayores para enfermedades como la artritis reumatoidea.

Hemos observado que el diflunisal es tan eficaz como la combinación de dextropropoxifeno y paracetamol (distalgesic, darvocet N) que se usa mucho como analgésico. Es también equivalente a la pentazocina. Una comparación con oxifenbutazona que hemos visto sugiere que el diflunisal puede ser algo superior. Otros estudios comparándolo con el fosfato de codeína, el dextropropoxifeno y la glafenina también parecen indicar que el diflunisal es superior. En muchas comparaciones más con la aspirina para diversas indicaciones se muestra que el diflunisal es superior, sobre todo en casos de artrosis, artritis reumatoidea y en la amplia variedad de dolores que se presentan en medicina general.

Apenas se sabe nada de los efectos secundarios probablemente debido a que no hay tantos. En mi experiencia, he tenido unos pocos casos de náusea y otros síntomas gastrointestinales diversos, incluyendo diarrea, pero según los trabajos presentados en el simposio está claro que la incidencia total de efectos secundarios es extremadamente baja. En comparación con la aspirina, hay menos repercusiones gástricas y el tinitus y la sordera no han creado problemas en relación con las dosis usadas. Se han presentado pruebas de que este medicamento es muy seguro. No parece

---

Diflunisal: Royal Society of Medicine International Congress and Symposium Series No. 6, published jointly by Academic Press Inc. (London) Ltd., and the Royal Society of Medicine.

provocar reacciones importantes y puede administrarse con warfarin. Cuando se comienza el diflunisal en pacientes que están tomando warfarin, se debe medir diariamente el tiempo de protrombina durante los primeros días. El diflunisal no causa hemorragia gastrointestinal oculta y es bueno saber que se puede aliviar el dolor y beber alcohol al mismo tiempo. Se han estudiado las intoxicaciones por dosis excesiva y este punto es muy importante para un medicamente que puede llegar a utilizarse ampliamente como analgésico y que el paciente dejará en el botiquín del cuarto de baño. Muchos analgésicos son bastante peligrosos en dosis excesivas, pero la experiencia preliminar sugiere que el diflunisal es más seguro a ese respecto.

Las informaciones comunicadas en este simposio sugieren que el diflunisal puede ser muy útil como otra preparación para aliviar el dolor. Supongo que, debido a su acción prolongada, será muy útil para pacientes que necesitan un tratamiento intenso y la administración regular de un analgésico. Para aquellos que necesitan un tratamiento intenso, creo que servirá muy bien para el tratamiento del lumbago, esguinces y desgarraduras y lesiones de varios tipos, o sea enfermedades que duran desde unos pocos días a algunas semanas. Para la administración continua será de utilidad en diversas enfermedades artríticas crónicas y en pacientes con dolores de cáncer.

A corrente posição do Diflunisal

E. C. HUSKISSON

St Bartholomew's Hospital, London, England

É evidente que o diflunisal é um composto muito diferente do seu ilustre antepassado, a aspirina, da qual foi derivado por um brilhante artifício de manipulação molecular. Em primeiro lugar, tem uma longa semi-vida, o que permite a administração duas vezes por dia e talvez produza alívio da dor durante toda a noite. Em segundo lugar, é um pouco mais eficaz do que a aspirina, talvez em resultado da florinação da molécula de aspirina. Em terceiro lugar, não causa zumbidos nem surdez, e pode ser de maior segurança do que a aspirina. O diflunisal não produz o mesmo efeito sobre as plaquetas que a aspirina, não provoca micro-hemorragias gástricas, e não tem causado acidose metabólica nos poucos casos de dose excessiva reportados até à data, e não causa as alterações hepáticas que por vezes ocorrem com a aspirina. A segurança e tolerância do composto talvez estejam relacionadas com a remoção do grupo acetil da aspirina.

Neste simpósio, viram-se provas evidentes de que o diflunisal é eficaz contra dores da região sacro-lombar, osteo-artrite, dores post-operatórias, dores de dentes, entorses e distensões musculares, artrite reumatóide e dores cancerosas. Tem definitivamente uma acção prolongada, e tem provado ser superior, durante um período de oito horas, a outros analgésicos de acção menos duradoura. Parece que a dose necessária é de 250 a 500 mg duas vezes por dia, sendo de prever que as doses maiores serão requeridas em condições como as de artrite reumatóide.

Viu-se que o diflunisal é tão eficaz como a combinação de dextropropoxifeno e paracetamol (Distalgesic, Darvocet N) que é largamente usada como um simples analgésico. Também é equivalente à pentazocina. Viu-se uma comparação com oxifenbutazona, que sugere que o diflunisal talvez seja um pouco superior. Vimos estudos comparando-o com fosfato de codeína, dextropropoxifeno e glafenina, mostrando uma vez mais que o diflunisal é superior. Vimos várias comparações com a aspirina em diferentes indicações, todas elas mostrando que o diflunisal é superior. Isto foi demonstrado em casos de osteo-artrite, artrite reumatóide, e ainda numa grande variedade de dores encontradas em clínica geral.

Muito pouco foi dito sobre efeitos secundários, talvez simplesmente porque não há muitos. Na minha experiência, tenho encontrado alguns casos de náusea e várias outras queixas gastro-intestinais, incluindo diarreia, mas vê-se claramente dos artigos apresentados neste simpósio que a incidência global de efeitos secundários com esta droga é extremamente baixa. Comparado com a aspirina, há menos efeitos gástricos, e zumbidos ou surdez não têm sido um problema às doses usadas até agora. Foi apresentada evidência de que esta droga é extremamente segura. Não parece produzir inter-reacções importantes, podendo ser administrada concomitantemente com a warfarin. Deve, contudo, ter-se certo cuidado quando se começa a dar diflunisal a um doente que ande a tomar warfarin, devendo medir-se diàriamente o tempo de protrombina durante os primeiros dias. O diflunisal não causa hemorragias ocultas gastro-intestinais, e é agradável saber que se pode aliviar dores e poder ao mesmo tempo beber bebidas alcoólicas. Os riscos de ingestão de doses excessivas têm sido discutidos, e é sem dúvida um assunto muito importante para uma droga que vai ser largamente usada, e vai ser deixada à mão em armários de casas de banho. Muitas das drogas que são usadas como analgésicos são, na realidade, bastante perigosas em dose excessiva, mas experiências preliminares sugerem que o diflunisal talvez seja mais seguro sobre este aspecto.

Experiências relatadas neste simpósio sugerem que o diflunisal será uma útil adição à lista de drogas já existentes para tratamento e alívio de dor. Eu penso que, devido à sua acção prolongada, ele será particularmente útil para doentes que necessitam um período de tratamento analgésico, ou a sua administração crónica. Para os que necessitem um limitado período de tratamento, creio que será particularmente útil no tratamento de dores sacro-lombares, entorses e distensões musculares, e outros tipos de injúrias corporais—doenças que duram alguns dias ou semanas. Para administração crónica, será de utilidade em várias doenças artríticas crónicas e em doentes com dores de etiologia cancerosa.